Medical Therapy in Glaucoma

Documenta Ophthalmologica
Proceedings Series volume 12

Editor H. E. Henkes

Dr. W. Junk bv Publishers The Hague 1977

Symposium on Medical Therapy in Glaucoma
Amsterdam, May 15, 1976

Edited by E. L. Greve

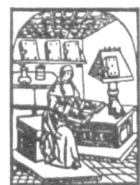

Dr. W. Junk bv Publishers The Hague 1977

Cover design: Max Velthuijs

© Dr W. Junk b.v. Publishers 1977
Softcover reprint of the hardcover 1st edition 1977

ISBN-13: 978-94-010-1311-6   e-ISBN-13: 978-94-010-1309-3
DOI: 10.1007/978-94-010-1309-3

CONTENTS

PREFACE

The proceedings of this symposium on Medical Therapy in Glaucoma are divided in four major parts.

The pharmacological introduction gives the reader a short description of factors that are involved between administration of the drug and its action at the desired position in the eye. The new and exciting field of drug delivery systems will be dealt with in this part and part II.

Originally we had asked Ken Richardson to give part of the lectures on Membrane technology and basic aspects of cholinergic action. Unfortunately at the last moment he could not come. Our thanks go to Gavin Paterson and Klaus Heilmann who were willing to take over a part of his job. Part II on cholinergic action offers next to the well-known drugs information about Ocusert.

Part III covers the new developments in the adrenergic field, including guanethidine and atenolol.

The clinical aspects of medical therapy in glaucoma are covered by Part IV.

Many subjects could not be handled. We left out the systemic treatment of glaucoma (diamox, mannitol etc.). We left out all special cases and problem cases. Some questions could be answered during the round table discussion, most remained unanswered. It is clear that there is enough subject-matter and interest for another symposium on therapy of glaucoma.

We thank Professors Crone and Bleeker for their help as chairmen of the sessions. Our thanks go to the invited speakers who gave such a clear and good presentation of their expert knowledge.

We are grateful to the support of Dr. Hoof of Grünenthal and Mr. Simons of Pharbil.

Mr. W.H. Miller and Miss E. Mutsaerts assisted in the organization.

We appreciate the pleasant and active cooperation of the publishers Dr. W. Junk B.V. and the stimulating enthousiasm of Professor Henkes, editor in chief of the Documenta Ophthalmologica Proceedings Series.

E.L. Greve & C.L. Dake

INTRODUCTION

C.L. DAKE & E.L. GREVE

(Amsterdam)

This symposium was organized to provide the general ophthalmologist with recent knowledge about medical therapy in glaucoma. We were pleasantly suprised that over 300 participants registered for this symposium. It shows that the management of glaucoma patients is of considerable interest to the general ophthalmologist.

At the moment it seems highly probable that increased IOP influences the vascular supply of the posterior part of the eye and in particular of the optic disc. This results in diminished perfusion pressure and sooner or later, depending on the height of the IOP and the state of the vessels nourishing the optic disc, damage to the optic nerve will become apparent. It can be expected that the susceptibility of the optic nerve head to IOP will differ in different persons, depending on the role of these two factors. And it is reasonable to assume that this susceptibility can change with time in the same person, depending on his or her age, general condition, vascular status, systemic hyper- or hyoptension, diabetes etc.

As yet there are no simple methods to measure perfusion flow in the posterior part of the eye, nor do we have objective methods to define what is called the critical pressure; the level of the IOP that gives rise to damage of the optic nerve head. The visual field is still our only, be it subjective, guide.

At present it is not possible to judge the results, if there are any, of measures that increase the resistance of the optic nerve tissue against the effect of raised IOP.

The treatment of glaucoma is therefore generally directed to attempts to lower IOP and to maintain the IOP at a level that supposedly prevents deterioration of the visual field. However, a deterioration of the visual field is a retrospective matter.

While IOP is mainly dependent on secretion of aqueous and resistance to outflow, lowering of IOP can be achieved by increasing the outflow or diminishing the secretion or both. How this can be effected by medical means was the subject of this symposium. We hope that it has increased the understanding of the medical management of the glaucoma patient.

FACTORS INFLUENCING THE CONCENTRATIONS OF A DRUG AT ITS SITE OF ACTION IN THE EYE

G. PATERSON

(London)

One considerable advantage in the administration of drugs in ocular therapy is the apparent accessibility of the target organ. It is generally a therapeutic aim to be able to achieve a high local concentration of a drug without having to suffer the disadvantages inherent in systemic administration. At times these disadvantages may be more imagined than real, but in the majority of instances the local effect sought, if generated throughout the body, would be catastrophic. So that the ophthalmologist takes recourse to a variety of means of local administration of drugs by topical application, by subconjunctival or retrobulbar injection, by iontophoresis, or by intra-cameral or intravitreous injection. Each of these modes of administration has been designed to localise an effective concentration of the drug at a specific site or sites.

TOPICAL APPLICATION

The cornea presents a formidable barrier to the absorption of drugs from the conjunctival sac. This is because of the anatomical structure of the cornea, and the nature of the applied drug. The cornea can be considered to be constructed of three layers, the epithelium and endothelium readily penetrated by fat-soluble substances, but not by electrolytes, and a third layer, the corneal stroma, through which electrolytes pass freely, but not fat-soluble material.

Most drugs applied topically to the eye are solutions of salts with most of the drug present in an ionised form. In this form the drug is unable to pass through the lipid barrier of the corneal epithelium. However, depending on the pH of the tear fluid and the pK_a of the drug a proportion of the drug will exist as the un-ionised form and will diffuse through the epithelium into the corneal stroma where it meets a medium which is essentially aqueous in nature. To diffuse through to the endothelium the drug must resume its ionised state only to meet up with a second lipid barrier, the endothelial layer, less impenetrable than the epithelium, but still demanding that the drug should alter its form to the un-ionised state before allowing it to pass into the aqueous humour. An example of the slow rate of penetration of an ionised substance through the undamaged cornea is fluorescein made use of extensively in ophthalmology. This will diffuse very slowly through the epithelium, unless this structure is damaged in some way, thus affording access to the stroma, where the fluorescein can diffuse and stain rapidly.

3

Subconjunctival injection

This means of injection by-passes the epithelial barrier, so that a drug can diffuse rapidly in high concentration in all directions in the stroma. A full comparison between the efficacy of this method and that of topical application is difficult, but subconjunctival application allows a greater degree of precision in localisation which justifies its use in particular instances where this is of prime importance. It is difficult to achieve satisfactory tissue levels with some antibiotics in the emergency management of acute infections of the anterior segment by routes other than subconjunctival injection. The disadvantages of the injection might then be outweighed by its advantages (Havener, 1974). Holland et al (1973) investigating the sensitising effect of chemical sympathectomy with 6-hydroxydopamine, used the technique of perilimbal subconjunctival injection of the drug. 6-Hydroxydopamine acts by destroying adrenergic nerves and in so doing increases the effectiveness of many sympathomimetic drugs. It was found by these authors that injections into the superior limbus had to be deliberately omitted, because diffusion of the drug to adrenergic nerves innervating the levator palpebrae muscles resulted in ptosis, indicating the effective diffusion of this drug after subconjunctival injection.

Retrobulbar or sub-Tenon injection

In glaucoma therapy these forms of injection are not used, since access to structures in the anterior chamber is minimal. Their usefulness is confined to localising drugs to sites of action at the posterior pole of the eye.

Iontophoresis

Drugs which ionise readily in aqueous solution can be carried through relatively impermeable barriers by a form of facilitated diffusion known as iontophoresis. In this method an electrode of the same charge as the drug ion is placed in contact with a solution of the drug, usually in a plastic eye cup covering the cornea, or on a cotton pad positioned according to the site of penetration. A second electrode of opposite charge is located at a distal area and a small current passed. This method has been used successfully by Kitazawa (1973, 1975) to convey 6-hydroxydopamine into the anterior chamber, thus minimising diffusion of the drug to unwanted sites.

This means of drug application has the inherent disadvantage of complexity of administration, and has received limited acceptance, and then mainly for special applications.

Systemic administration of drugs

By this means drugs have to diffuse in the bloodstream before reaching the eye, and, consequently, side effects irrelevant to ocular effects may have to be accepted. In the case of acetazolamide, topical application is ineffective in lowering IOP, and oral or intravenous administration is used, the latter route principally in the treatment of acute glaucoma. A more recent addition to glaucoma therapy, the beta-adrenoceptor blocking agents, are also very effective ocular hypotensive agents given orally, although in some recent trials some of these drugs have also been shown to have considerable effect after topical application. (Bucci et al., 1968, Phillips et al., 1967, Vale et al., 1972).

Distribution and fate of drugs after absorption

When a drug enters the anterior chamber, the rate of turnover of aqueous humour to a large extent dictates its duration of action, since the concentration of drug in the aqueous will act as a reservoir for renewal of concentrations at active sites. In the regions bathed by the aqueous humour the drug will be subjected to metabolic pathways designed to remove or modify both naturally-occurring and foreign substances. One such pathway is the uptake mechanism in the cell membrane of adrenergic nerve terminals which removes noradrenaline and adrenaline when these are in close proximity to the terminals. This mechanism − known as $Uptake_1$ − is the physiological means by which the body terminates adrenergic nerve activity, at the same time conserving the noradrenaline for future release. When either adrenaline or noradrenaline is applied topically to the conjunctival sac, the applied concentration must be at least 0.5 per cent. to achieve an appreciable fall in intra-ocular pressure of adequate duration. It would appear that much of the absorbed drug is removed by adrenergic nerves, since if the $Uptake_1$ mechanism is inhibited by drugs, protriptyline (Langham & Carmel, 1968) or guanethidine (Paterson & Paterson, 1972) or if the nerves are destroyed either by chronic denervation after superior cervical ganglionectomy (Sears & Sherk, 1963) or by chemical sympathectomy with 6-hydroxydopamine (Holland et al., 1973) the effectiveness of the adrenaline or noradrenaline is increased manyfold. The supersensitivity achieved by the uptake inhibitors is not as great as that seen after either form of sympathectomy (Kitazawa, 1975, Sears & Sherk, 1963). This is probably related to two features, first, the greater effectiveness of the sympathectomy procedures, where the nerves are completely removed, and, second, the non-specific sensitisation seen after nerve removal, which is independent of uptake mechanisms. In this connection Holland & Wei (1973) reported an increased lowering of IOP with isoprenaline (a catecholamine not taken up by adrenergic nerves) in patients subjected to ocular chemical sympathectomy with 6-hydroxydopamine.

NEWER FORMS OF DRUG ADMINISTRATION

A promising advance in drug delivery is the development of the membrane controlled delivery unit (Ocusert® P20) where the drug, to begin with pilocarpine, is held in a central core within a flexible envelope of a synthetic polymer (Armaly & Rao, 1974, Richardson, 1975). The pilocarpine is then released slowly into tear fluid then to be absorbed in the usual way. A great advantage of this method is the constancy of release of pilocarpine, said to be in the region of 20 micrograms per hour. This means of administration has its counterpart in a continuous infusion system used to administer pilocarpine in a comparison of this method with the conventional single drop (Birmingham et al., 1976). It was possible with the continuous perfusion to use a much weaker solution of pilocarpine.

REFERENCES

Armaly, M.F. & Rao, K.R. The effect of Pilocarpine Ocuserts on Ocular Pressure. In: Leopold, I.H. (Ed.): Symposium on Ocular Therapy, St. Louis, The C.V. Mosby Company. (1974).

Birmingham, A.T., Bedford, G., Galloway, N.R., Spencer, S.A. & Walker, D.A. Continuous Infusion of the Conjunctival Sac in Normal Subjects and Patients with Chronic Glaucoma. *Trans. Ophthal. Soc. U.K.* 00: – (1976).

Bucci, M.G., Giraldi, J.P., Missiroli, A. & Virno, M. Local Administration of Propranolol in the Glaucoma Therapy. *Boll. Ocul.* 47: *51*, (1968).

Havener, W.H. Ocular Pharmacology. 3rd. Edition. St. Louis, The C.V. Mosby Company. (1974).

Holland, M.G. & Wei, C. Chemical Sympathectomy in Glaucoma: An Investigation of Alpha and Beta Adrenergic Supersensitivity. *Ann. Ophthal.* 5: *783-796* (1973).

Holland, M.G., Wei, C. & Gupta, S. Review and Evaluation of 6-Hydroxydopamine (6-HD): Chemical Sympathectomy for the Treatment of Glaucoma. *Ann. Ophthal.* 5: *539-558* (1973).

Kitazawa, Y. Discussion on the Pharmacology of the Adrenergic Therapy of Glaucoma. In: Etienne, R. & Paterson, G.D. (Eds.) International Glaucoma Symposium, Albi. Marseille, Diffusion Générale de Librairie. (1975).

Kitazawa, Y., Nose, H. & Horie, T. The Effects of Chemical Sympathectomy on Intra-Ocular Pressure in Human Subjects. *Acta Soc. Ophthal. Japan,* 77, *1901-1907* (1973).

Langham, M.E. The Pharmacology of the Adrenergic Therapy of Glaucoma. In: Etienne, R. & Paterson, G.D. (Eds.) International Glaucoma Symposium, Albi. Marseille, Diffusion Générale de Librairie. (1975).

Langham, M.E. & Carmel, D. The Action of Protriptyline on Adrenergic Mechanisms In Rabbit, Primate and Human Eyes. *J. Pharmac. exp. Ther.,* 163, *368* (1968).

Paterson, G.D. & Paterson, G. Drug Therapy of Glaucoma. *Brit. J. Ophthal.* 56, *288-294* (1972).

Paterson, G.D., Paterson, G. & Miller, S.J.H. The Non-Miotic Treatment of Open Angle Glaucoma. In: Etienne, R & Paterson, G.D. (Eds.) International Glaucoma Symposium, Albi. Marseille, Diffusion Générale de Librairie.

Phillips, C.I., Howitt, G. & Rowlands, D.J. Propranolol as Ocular Hypotensive Agent. *Brit. J. Ophthal.* 51, *222* (1967).

Richardson, K.T. Ocular Microtherapy Zero Order Drug Release. In: Etienne, R. & Paterson, G.D. (Eds.). International Glaucoma Symposium, Albi. Marseille, Diffusion Générale de Librairie.

Sears, M.L. & Sherk, T.E. Supersensitivity of the Aquous Outflow Resistance in Rabbits after Sympathetic Denervation. *Nature* 197, *387* (1963).

Vale, J., Gibbs, A.C.C. & Phillips, C.I. Topical Propranolol and Ocular Tension in the Human. *Brit. J. Ophthal.* 56, *770* (1972).

Author's address:
Department of Pharmacology
University of London
King's College
Strand, London WC2
England

MEMBRANE TECHNOLOGY
PRINCIPLES AND THERAPEUTIC POSSIBILITIES
OF CONTROLLED DELIVERY OF DRUGS

K. HEILMANN

(Munich)

The introduction of the first examples of Therapeutic Systems in Europe — Ocusert® for delivering drugs to the eye and Biograviplan® designed to release progesterone into the uterine cavity and to provide a contraceptive effect (Chemie Gruenenthal GmbH, Stolberg, Federal Republic of Germany) — has because of lacking knowledge frequently led to misunderstandings which were intensified by an undiscriminating discussion on the costs associated with the application of some of these systems.

The process of drug formulation was for centuries the secret and art of the pharmacists, it was later taken over by the pharmaceutical industry and today lies almost exclusively in their hands. The pharmaceutical industry has, in the last few decades developed an impressing arsenal of new chemical compounds, many of which have become effective drugs. In contrast to the prodigious and successful, albeit costly struggles to synthesise new substances are the relatively modest efforts to develop new types of dosage forms.

A pharmacologically active substance is not necessarily an effective drug. In order to attain rational drug therapy on a higher level, it is no longer sufficient merely to know the molecular structure of a drug. In the last few years especially, efforts have been intensified to characterise pharmacologically active substances pharmacokinetically too*. In this way it is possible to establish quantitative relationships between the pharmacological effects of a substance and its concentration in body tissues. To use informations gained from such basic research also in therapy, it is necessary in many cases to optimize patterns and portals of drug administration. Therapeutic Systems represent an absolutely new beginning in this connection; the principles and therapeutic possibilities of controlled delivery of drugs are briefly reported here.

Therapeutic systems vs. conventional dosage forms

A Therapeutic System is a drug-containing device or dosage form that ad-

---

* Pharmacokinetics is that branch of pharmacology that studies the relationship between rate of drug administration and the concentration of drug in plasma or other body fluids and also tries to define the rates at which drug levels first build up and then decline following drug administration.

7

ministers one or more drugs at a programmed rate, at a specified body site, for a prescribed period of time (Zaffaroni, 1971). The purpose of a Therapeutic System is to provide continuous supervision of drug therapy and to maintain this control over extended periods of time. If Therapeutic Systems are compared with conventional dosage forms, it is necessary to point out the limits of effectiveness of conventional drugs. These limitations have their origin in the formulation of a substance and are closely associated with the patient himself who is responsible for the proper carrying out of the prescribed regimen. It is a characteristic of self-administered conventional dosage forms that only a relatively short duration can be attained with them, so that in order to prevent sawtooth pattern of drug delivery and its reflection in drug concentrations in body fluids and tissues, the frequency of administration must be raised. This is not without problems, because toxic effects may appear with over-dosage. The limited duration of action is directly connected with the characteristic delivery pattern of almost all conventional dosage forms: initially, increased amounts of the drug are given up to surrounding tissues at time varying rates and decline continually thereafter. A period of over-dosage alternates with a period of under-dosage, and for only a relatively short time an optimal concentration is maintained. Among others the pharmaceutical industry has always been conscious of the narrow frequency range of self-administered drugs, but had sought the solution in prolonging the half-life of drug molecules in the body to achieve a reduction of dosage frequency.

Closely connected with the narrow frequency range of most conventional drugs is the patients limited reliability to follow a prescribed regimen. Particularly when drugs must be taken for years, and therefore in the treatment of chronic diseases especially, a waning of the patient's cooperation is striking. In various studies carried out independently of each other in Europe and the USA, it was found that the prescribed regimen was not followed by about 30 to 40% of patients. Faulty compliance is the rule rather than the exception. It was also established that the individual doctor is not conscious of this situation and considers such results to be inapplicable to him and his patients. In this respect illusionistic thoughts seem to be widespread among physicians!

The realisation of the concept of controlled drug delivery starts from the idea that such a goal will not be reached by manipulating drug molecules but that the phase of drug release from the dosage form must be influenced. With the help of modern technology a new class of dosage forms with controlled and constant release of a drug was developed. In contrast to conventional first-order dosage forms, in Therapeutic Systems the drug is released in a zero-order pattern: the need for an initial overdosage does not arise and significantly smaller amounts of substance are required to obtain completely continuous and effective drug levels. For the future it is especially interesting that even drugs with a short biological half-life can now be used which previously had to remain unused for therapy.

A Therapeutic System consists of four major components: the drug or drugs; a drug delivery module; a platform and the therapeutic programme.

The drug delivery module is located in the platform. It is responsible for the release of the drug according to the determined therapeutic programme and consists of four elements: the drug reservoir; the rate controller; the energy source and the delivery portal.

The materials used for the drug delivery module are synthetic. Synthetic polymer membranes are characterised both by their solubility and by their density, for which reason they can be adapted to almost all therapeutic programmes. The platform also consists of synthetic biocompatible materials which must be so designed that the system can be easily and safely used by the patient himself. For achieving controlled drug release, mechanical, chemical or electrochemical energy can be utilized.

Therapeutic Systems are principally differentiated as open- and closed-loop systems. In the following open-loop systems are discussed, which are designed both for local and systemic use.

Therapeutic systems for local use

Ocular Therapeutic System

The first examples of Therapeutic Systems were those developed for the use in the eye. They are differentiated into 'Diffusion units', 'Osmotic units'

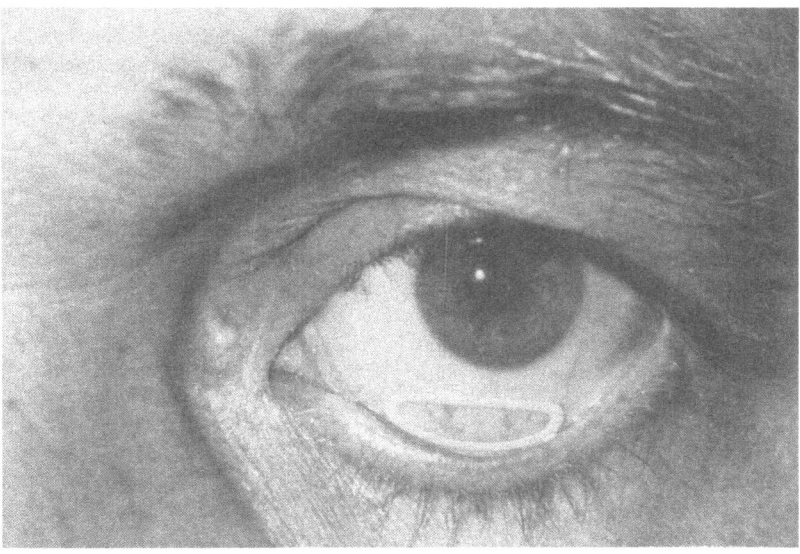

Fig. 1. Diffusion unit Ocusert. The physical properties of Ethylene-vinyl-acetate (EVA) copolymer provide great flexibility, clarity and selective permeability. The white border around the unit is provided by EVA impregnated with titanium dioxide. The elliptically shaped Ocusert remains within the cul-de-sac day and night over a period of one week.

Thanks are due to Ferdinand Enke Verlag, Stuttgart, for permission to reproduce this figure (from: Therapeutische Systeme. Konzept und Realisation organspezifischer Arzneiverabreichung, by Klaus Heilmann, 1977).

9

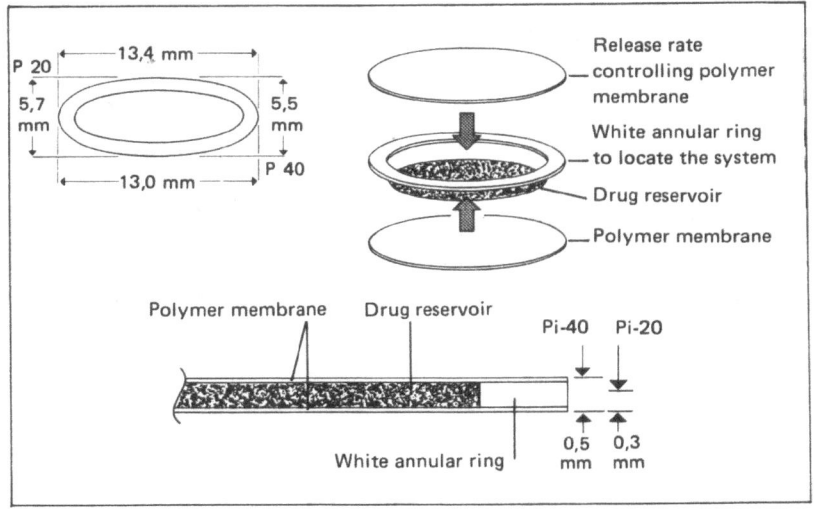

Fig. 2. Ocusert design. The EVA copolymer membrane serves not only as drug reservoir for pilocarpine but also as the rate-controlling membrane and delivery portal.

Thanks are due to Ferdinand Enke Verlag, Stuttgart, for permission to reproduce this figure (from: Therapeutische Systeme. Konzept und Realisation organspezifischer Arzneiverabreichung, by Klaus Heilmann, 1977).

and 'Erodible units'; two types of osmotic units are designed: the 'Mini-pump unit' and the 'Micro-compartment unit'. (fig. 1, 2 and 3)

The unit available under the name Ocusert works on the diffusion principle; it is at present obtainable with pilocarpine and later will also be available with epinephrine/pilocarpine and with carbachol for the treatment of glaucoma. With the diffusion unit a constant drug release over a period of seven days is possible. Besides what is probably the most important therapeutic field-chronic open-angle glaucoma-, the various units are suitable for the treatment of bacterial and viral infections of the eye, cortisone treatment being able to enter a new era through the zero-order release pattern, and for endemic diseases (trachoma), for which there are suitable drugs but so far no suitable dosage forms to treat these diseases effectively.

Uterine Therapeutic System

Biograviplan represents a new class of contraceptive devices. Biograviplan is a T-shaped unit which is placed in the uterine cavity and is effective as a contraceptive for one year. Progesterone is stored in crystalline form within the unit, the natural pregnancy hormone is used locally for the first time; the one-year's store of hormone is 38 mg, a total of 24 mg is delivered into the uterine cavity by diffusion in 365 days, with a constant rate of 65 µg/day. Progesterone has a short half-life, is already rapidly decomposed in the upper layers of the endometrium and metabolised there to

10

substances with no endocrine activity. With regard to the increasing discussion on the side effects of oral contraceptives it is important to indicate that with the Therapeutic System Biograviplan no systemic hormone effect occurs.

Therapeutic systems for systemic use

Liquid Infusion System

Interesting and very promising aspects are offered by an infusion system (Liquid Infusion System AR/MED®, Alza Corp., Palo Alto, Calif.). The drug in liquid formulation is stored under pressure and continuously delivered into the blood circulation. The light weight unit (45 g when empty) is worn on the arm and includes non-collapsible tubing, micro-needle, bacterial filter and warning system. The drug is placed in cartridges which are changed by the patient himself, the drug release rate being adjustable by the doctor exclusively. The drug delivery is metered through an adjustable, precalibrated precision valve making it possible to infuse drugs for weeks and months. Thus a reliable and safe therapy can be carried out without the patient being admitted to hospital. This also saves hospital expenses, because up to now infusion therapy meant hospitalization. The system was first clinically tested in patients who required continuous administration of heparin as an anticoagulant and prolonged treatment of cancer chemotherapy.

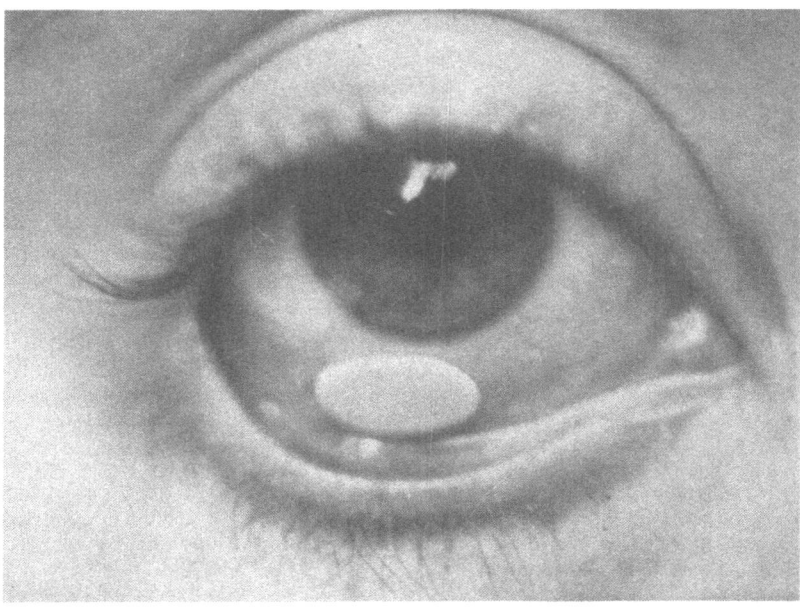

Fig. 3. Ocular Therapeutic System: Example of an 'Osmotic Unit' ('Minipump-Unit').

11

Oral Osmotic Therapeutic System

A new approach in oral drug therapy is the membrane-controlled Thera-peutic System Oros (Alza Corp., Palo Alto, Calif.). It resembles a conven-tional tablet, stores the drug in solid form and delivers it in solution. The platform is inert and is excreted after the functional life of the system is ended. The osmotic activity of the drug causes water to be transferred from the intestinal lumen through the semipermeable membrane into the system; the resulting hydrostatic pressure rise causes delivery of a saturated solution. The release rate is therefore predictable and constant; drugs with short half-lifes or such damaging the gastro-intestinal tract if released too quickly can be used. Considerably smaller amounts of drug may be necessary to produce the same therapeutic effect in comparison to conventional dosage forms. This means a reduction of undesirable side effects at the same time.

Transdermal Therapeutic System

The Transdermal Therapeutic System (ALZA Corp., Palo Alto, Calif.), un-like the infusion system, enables a drug to act systemically without penetra-tion of the skin by a needle. The drug is transferred through the intact skin

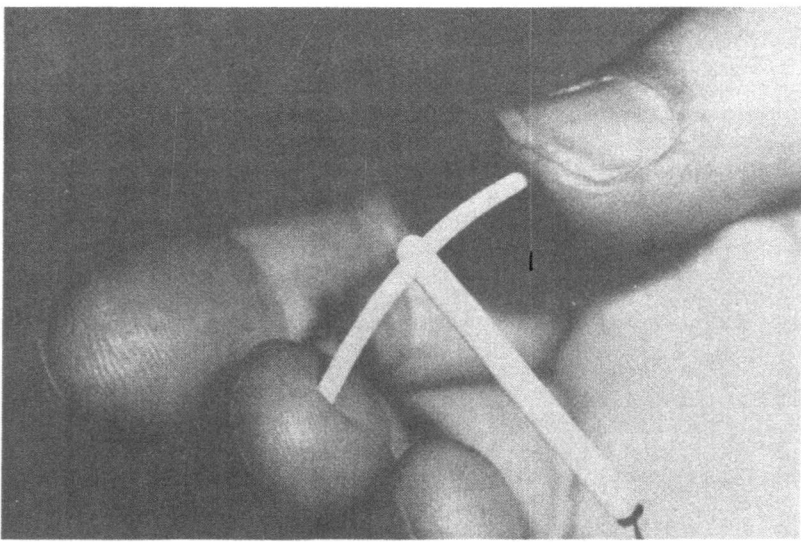

Fig. 4. Uterine Therapeutic System Biograviplan® (Progestasert®). The T-shaped unit has to be placed in the uterine cavity. The figure shows the size and the flexibility of the unit. Biograviplan is a diffusion unit and stores Progesterone for one year. The constant delivery rate is 65 μg/day.

Thanks are due to Ferdinand Enke Verlag, Stuttgart, for permission to reproduce this figure (from: Therapeutische Systeme, Konzept und Realisation organspezifischer Arzneiverabreichung by Klaus Heilmann, 1977).

by diffusion. The unit is similar to a piece of plaster, is applicated to a selected skin surface (retro-auricular or scapular region) and releases the drug at a constant rate. The system was first designed for scopolamine − an effective antinauseant − and used for the prophylaxis and treatment of motion sickness. Scopolamine is the most suitable substance for this purpose, but up to now it could not be used in conventional dosage form because of too severe general side effects; antihistamine preparations had to be used instead. With the aid of the Transdermal Therapeutic System, the use of scopolamine with a significant reduction of systemic effects has become successful. At the present time, attempts are being made to use the system for the treatment of high blood pressure.

CONCLUSIONS

Because of the controlled drug release, Therapeutic Systems include the possibility of releasing the drug at an optimal rate at the selected target site and at the same time reducing to a minimum the tissue level in organs which must be exposed to the drug but in which no therapeutic effect is intended. Furthermore, numerous active pharmacological substances which previously

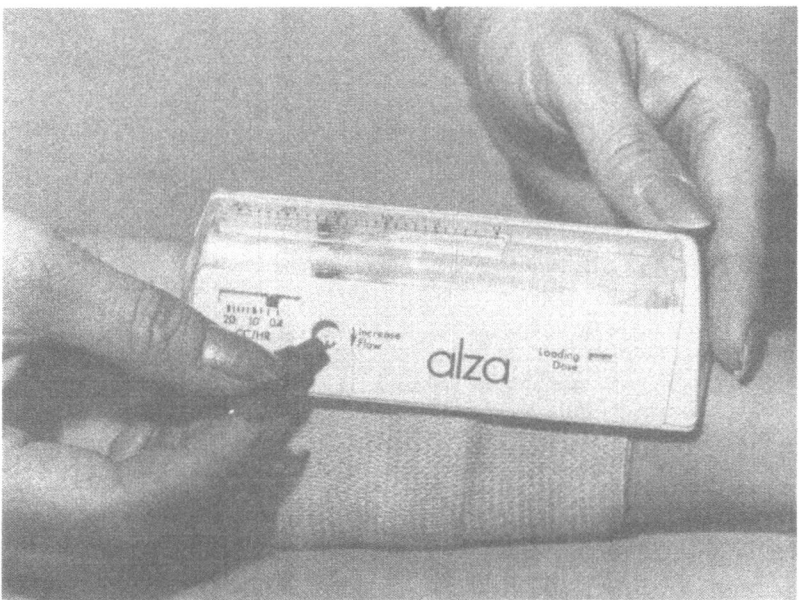

Fig. 5. Liquid infusion system AR/MED.® The figure shows the unit with the cartridge. The drug in liquid formulation is stored in the cartridge which can be changed by the patient himself.

Thanks are due to Ferdinand Enke Verlag, Stuttgart, for permission to reproduce this figure (from: Therapeutische Systeme. Konzept und Realisation organspezifischer Arzneiverabreichung, by Klaus Heilmann, 1977).

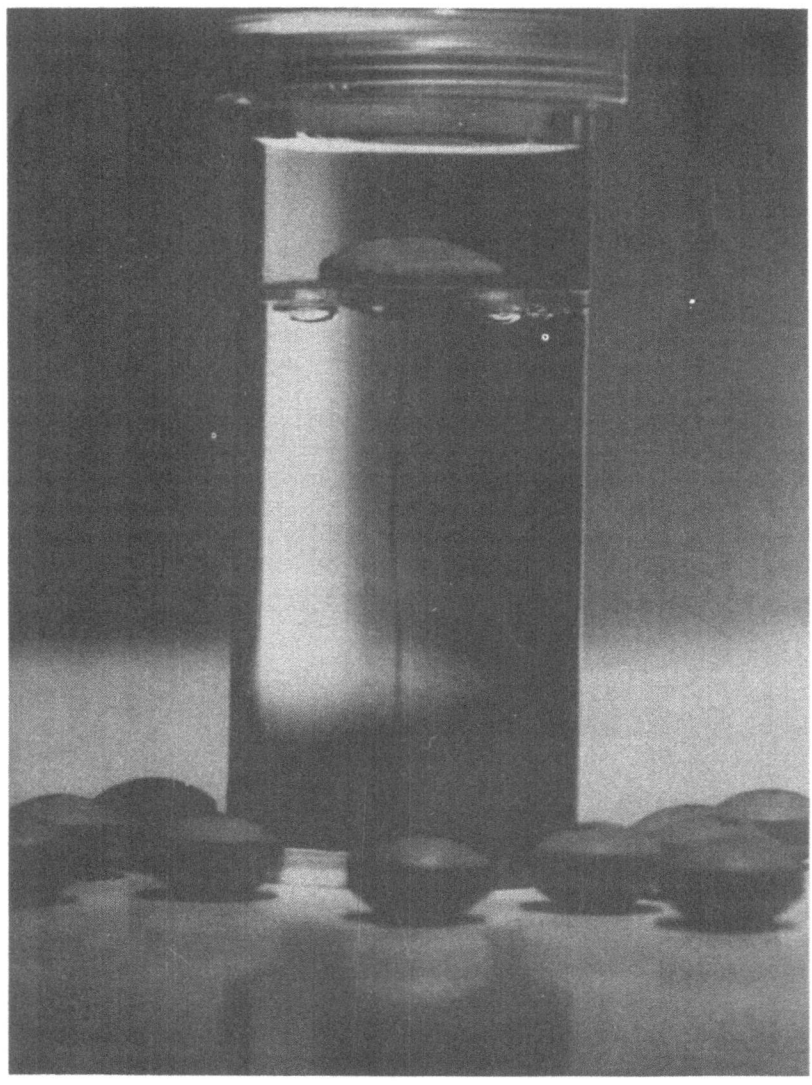

Fig. 6. Oral Osmotic Therapeutic System OROS®. The figure shows that OROS resembles a conventional tablet, which stores a drug in solid form and delivers it in solution. The model shows that the unit has one delivery portal.

Thanks are due to Ferdinand Enke Verlag, Stuttgart, for permission to reproduce this figure (from: Therapeutische Systeme, Konzept und Realisation organspezifischer Arzneiverabreichung, by Klaus Heilmann, 1977).

14

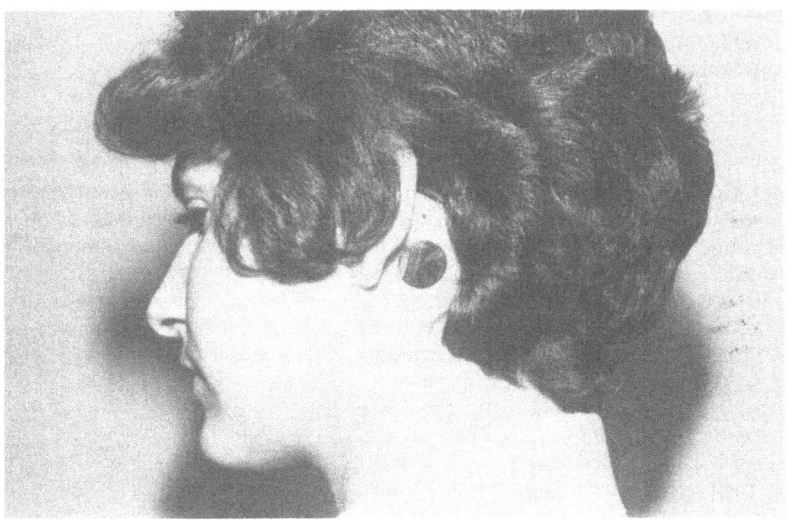

Fig. 7. A Transdermal Therapeutic System transfers a drug through the intact skin by diffusion. The unit resembles a piece of plaster which is applicated to the retro-auricular region.

could not be used because of their small therapeutic index or their short half-life, can now be introduced to therapy with Therapeutic Systems. Finally, frequent administration of a drug and supervision of the treatment by the patient himself is no longer necessary, because the system itself takes over this task with great precision.

The possibilities of Therapeutic Systems are not yet exhausted. Medical therapy, as everybody knows, cannot be standardised; individual differences in response to drugs are unusually great. A drug in a particular concentration has not the same effect in all persons. The factors which can influence the efficacy of drugs have only been investigated systematically in the last few years. Biological processes follow an inborn endogenous rhythm. We know today that paying attention to these endogenous rhythms, which may be disturbed by exogenous influences, is important in medical treatment. With Therapeutic Systems it is not only possible to release a drug constantly and controlled, it is also possible to programme particular time patterns of drug release so that the drug release can be adapted to endogenous rhythms.

Let it be said that wrong impressions must arise if the costs of therapeutics are compared in isolation; when comparing conventional dosage forms with Therapeutic Systems, a new class of dosage forms, it is essential to set the limited possibilities of conventional dosage forms against the therapeutic potential of Therapeutic Systems and to compare with each other the advantages and disadvantages for the patient.

The concept of a controlled delivery of drugs and the engineering development of Therapeutic Systems must be regarded as a milestone in the history of therapeutics which is comparable to discoveries like those of the antibiotics, the sulphonamides, the vitamins or steroids. I strongly believe that Therapeutic Systems will produce far-reaching changes in the pharmaceutical industry and in medicine within the next decade.

LITERATURE

Alza Corp.: The OCUSERT (pilocarpine) Pilo-20/Pilo-40 Ocular Therapeutic System. A new approach to treating ocular hypertension. A monograph. Palo Alto, 1974.

Heilmann, K.: Therapeutische Systeme. Konzept und Realisation organspezifischer Arzneiverabreichung. F. Enke, Stuttgart 1977.

Heilmann, K.: Therapeutic Systems. Conception and realization of membrane controlled drug delivery. Thieme Editious, G. Thieme, Stuttgart (1977, in press).

Heilmann, K.: Pharmacology. In: 'Glaucoma' (K. Heilmann and K.T. Richardson, eds.), G. Thieme, Stuttgart (1977, in press).

Richardson, K.T.: Ocular Microtherapy. Membrane-controlled drug delivery. *Arch. Ophthalmol.* 93, *74−86* (1975).

Richardson, K.T.: Membrane controlled drug delivery. In: 'Symposium on Glaucoma. Transactions of the New Orleans Academy of Ophthalmology' (D.R. Anderson, ed.), pp. 50-67. C.V. Mosby, St. Louis 1975.

Zaffaroni, A.: Therapeutic implications of controlled drug delivery. Presented at the 6th International Congress of Pharmacology, Helsinki 1975.

Author's address:
Hochkalterstrasse 8
D−8000 München
West Germany

THE ACTIONS AND USES OF PARASYMPATHOMIMETIC DRUGS IN GLAUCOMA

G. PATERSON

(London)

The parasympathetic nervous system and its manipulation by drugs have been associated now for a century, since the introduction of pilocarpine in 1876 by Weber. This drug, a directly-acting parasympathomimetic, has, despite its many drawbacks, maintained its front-line position in the ophthalmologist's armamentarium. Now, however, after this lapse of time during which many alternative therapeutic and surgical measures have appeared and (many) disappeared some of pilocarpine's drawbacks are now yielding to the advances in the modifications of delivery systems (see Heilmann, this symposium).

PARASYMPATHETIC INNERVATION OF OCULAR STRUCTURES

Post-ganglionic nerves make synaptic contact with many stuctures in the orbit. Supplies to the constrictor pupillae, the circular band of the ciliary muscle, and the longitudinal and meridional bands of the ciliary muscle are well established in anatomical and physiological terms. The position of innervation of the ciliary body processes by parasympathetic nerves is far from clear. Histologically, the presence of post-ganglionic cholinergic nerves in the ciliary processes has been shown, but the cellular elements innervated have not been determined. Parasympathetic stimulation is known to cause an initial rise in intra-ocular pressure which has been suggested to be due to a dilatation of intercellular spaces in the ciliary epithelium (Uusitalo, Stjernschantz & Palkama, 1974).

Methods used to identify cholinergic nerves and synapses are; 1. histochemical methods which depend upon the hydrolytic properties of neuronal and synaptic acetylcholinesterase, and 2. electron-microscopical and autoradiographic techniques, (1. Koelle & Friedenwald, 1949; 2. Uusitalo & Palkama, 1972).

CHOLINOCEPTOR DIFFERENTIATION

Acetylcholine is the functional neurotransmitter at all cholinergic nerve endings, but the junctions at which it acts can be separated on the basis of the pharmacological properties of the receptors located on the post-junctional membrane. One receptor form, for which muscarine was found to be a specific agonist and atropine a specific antagonist was described as 'muscarinic'. The second form, with which nicotine reacted specifically and which could be blocked by curare-like substances became known as 'nicotinic', (Dale, 1914). Muscarinic receptors are found at all parasympathetic and some sympathetic cholinergic post-ganglionic neuro-effector junctions and nicotinic receptors are located at all autonomic ganglionic synapses, the adrenal medulla and the skeletal neuromuscular junction.

It is with muscarinic receptors that most of the cholinergic therapy of glaucoma is concerned. It is still difficult to localize these receptors at the sites of action of parasympathomimetics, but the recent rapid advances in receptor isolation techniques make the prospect less remote (de Robertis, 1975).

ACTIONS OF PARASYMPATHOMIMETIC DRUGS

Drugs which mimic the action of parasympathetic nerve stimulation may do this in two ways. The can activate the receptors directly (Table 1) or they can inhibit junctional acetylcholinesterase, thus increasing the local concentration of acetylcholine (Table 2).

Table 1. Drugs which act as direct agonists at muscarinic receptors.
(Drugs in parenthesis are no longer in general ophthalmic use).

Pilocarpine
Carbachol
Aceclidine
(Bethanechol)
(Furmethide)
(Acetylcholine)
(Methacholine)

Table 2. Drugs which inhibit acetylcholinesterase so increasing local concentrations of acetylcholine. (Drugs in parenthesis are no longer in general ophthalmic use).

Reversible anticholinesterases
    (Edrophonium)
    (Eserine)
    (Neostigmine)
    (Pyridostigmine)
    Demecarium

Irreversible anticholinesterases
    Di-isopropyl phosphorofluoridate; DFP; dyflos
    Echothiophate
    (Tetraethyl pyrophosphate)
    (Diethyl-p-nitrophenyl phosphate; Mintacol)

DIRECT AGONISTS

Pilocarpine

It is a testimony to its effectiveness that this plant alkaloid has not been replaced by a suitable synthetic substitute. It has been investigated more than any other miotic drug, but its principal mode of action is still unclear. It reduces secretion of aqueous humour and increases outflow from the anterior chamber. These and other effects of pilocarpine such as miosis and spasm of accommodation are dissociable, (Törnqvist, 1964, 1967; Bárány, 1966; Barsam, 1972). Armaly & Rao, (1973) and Holland (1974) also found that pilocarpine released from 'Ocuserts' caused less miosis for the same fall in intra-ocular pressure than did the application of pilocarpine eye drops.

However, there are undoubtedly several sites of action of pilocarpine which contribute overall to the fall in intra-ocular pressure. A reduction in the secretion of aqueous humour from isolated ciliary processes of the rabbit has been described by Berggren (1965). Alm, Bill & Young (1973) studied blood flow through the anterior uvea in monkeys, using a blood flow technique employing radio-actively labelled microspheres and showed that pilocarpine was capable of increasing blood flow through the iris, ciliary processes and ciliary muscle by up to 200 per cent. At the same time blood flow through the retina and choroid was unaffected. It is likely that these last two vascular beds have no muscarinic receptors in their make-up.

The explanation most favoured for the increased facility of outflow of aqueous humour is that of an action of pilocarpine on the longitudinal bundle of the ciliary muscle, decreasing the resistance to outflow through the trabecular meshwork (Bárány, 1962, 1966). It is felt by many workers that the laminar arrangement of the trabecular meshwork dictates drainage through into the canal of Schlemm; any mechanical rearrangement of the spaces within the meshworks will then alter outflow (Grant, 1958, 1963; Dannheim & Bárány, 1969; Ellingson & Grant, 1971a, b; Peterson, Jocson & Sears, 1971). A role of the swelling and shrinkage of the endothelial cells lining the trabeculae has also been suggested (Tripathi, 1974). A further mechanism to be considered may be through some influence on the giant vacuoles which have been suggested to be the means of transport of the bulk outflow of aqueous humour from the anterior chamber (Tripathi, 1968, 1972, 1974). However, when pilocarpine is given intravenously it causes an immediate increase in outflow facility. This effect is at a maximum within two minutes and is suggested to be due to an action on ciliary muscle; any direct effect on trabecular structures would be ruled out since the concentration of pilocarpine in the aqueous would be too low for such an action (Bárány, 1967).

The effects of pilocarpine in each facet of its actions in the eye are dose-dependent (Törnqvist, 1964, 1967; Harris & Galin, 1970; Drance & Nash, 1971; Drance, Bensted & Schulzer, 1974), but there are major differences in the efficacy of the same concentration when compared on eyes with lightly or heavily pigmented irides (Harris & Galin, 1971; Barsam, 1972). Where the iris is heavily pigmented the effective concentration of pilocarpine must be increased to produce the same fall in intra-ocular pressure. Lyons & Krohn (1973) investigated pilocarpine uptake by pigmented and albino irides and ciliary bodies and found that the uptake by the pigmented tissues was two to three times greater than for the non-pigmented tissues. This uptake was unrelated to the enzymatic breakdown of pilocarpine which occurs in these tissues.

EFFECTS OF PILOCARPINE ON ACCOMMODATION

This is one of the irritating and disabling side effects of pilocarpine therapy, especially in young patients where the effect of the spasm of accommodation is several dioptres in magnitude. Even in presbyopes, however, a considerable change can occur, ranging from 2 to 13 dioptres (Abramson, Franzen & Coleman, 1973).

OTHER DIRECTLY-ACTING PARASYMPATHOMIMETICS

Aceclidine has been used with some success in chronic simple glaucoma (Lieberman & Leopold, 1967; Etienne, Barut & Gonzales-Bouchon, 1967; Demailly, 1968; Drance, Fairclough & Schulzer, 1972). However, there seems little difference between the effects of this drug and pilocarpine (Romano, 1970), although Fechner, Teichmann & Weyrauch (1975) claim that the fall in intra-ocular pressure is not associated with a change in accommodation. There may be some use for this drug in patients allergic to pilocarpine.

Carbachol is a carbamic acid ester of choline and because of this difference in structure from acetylcholine is resistant to hydrolysis by acetylcholinesterase. Its effect is more prolonged than that of pilocarpine, both in its miotic effect and in its ocular hypotensive action. Comparing a 0.75 per cent. solution of carbachol with a 2 per cent. solution of pilocarpine, the carbachol was more effective on both pupil diameter and intra-ocular pressure (O'Brien & Swan, 1942). However, carbachol causes more accommodative distress and headaches than pilocarpine. Also it is less well absorbed through the corneal epithelium and has to be administered with a wetting agent, benzalkonium.

ANTICHOLINESTERASE DRUGS

Most of these substances have no direct effect of their own and owe their activity to the build-up of acetylcholine which occurs after acetylcholinesterase has been inhibited (see Hobbiger, 1966). These drugs are sub-classified into two groups, the reversible and the irreversible anticholinesterases.

Reversible anticholinesterases

Eserine and neostigmine are ester derivatives of carbamic acid and after reacting with acetylcholinesterase they are hydrolysed by the enzyme, the carbamate moiety remaining bound to the enzyme. The cholinesterase is still inhibited at this stage, but the process enters a second, slower stage during which the enzyme-carbamate complex dissociates to regenerate the uninhibited enzyme. The duration of the action of a reversible anticholinesterase applied topically is from 12 to 36 hours and although this might suggest their use in the therapy of glaucoma, local side effects such as muscle twitching and systemic side effects have precluded their adoption.

Irreversible anticholinesterases

These are organophosphorus derivatives and react with acetylcholinesterase at its esteratic site. The phosphorylated enzyme has a very stable configuration and hydrolyses extremely slowly. Because of this, their duration of action is prolongued and they need only be administered at infrequent intervals, although they are generally applied daily.

The first of this group to be introduced was di-isopropylphosphorofluoridate (D.F.P.; dyflos) (Leopold & Comroe, 1946), but it suffered from the disadvantage that it had to be dissolved in an oily medium. Also it hydrolyses readily if contaminated with water. It has been supplanted by echothiophate (Leopold, Gold & Gold, 1957) and by mintacol (Glees & Wustenberg, 1949). Systemic absorption of these anticholinesterases presents a problem. Erythrocyte acetylcholinesterase and plasma cholinesterase are reduced to 50 per cent in activity after 4 weeks treatment topically with 0.06 per cent. echothiophate (Leopold, 1966). With this systemic absorption come the disadvantages of systemic side effects, but the most disturbing side effect is local and is not recorded with either pilocarpine or reversible anticholinesterase therapy. This is the induction of lens opacities in eyes where no previous history presented and the deterioration of the state of the lens where pretreatment opacities existed (Axelsson & Holmberg, 1966). Subsequent reports have confirmed these changes (Shaffer & Hetherington, 1966; de Roetth, 1966; Tarkkanen & Karjalainen, 1966). Levene (1969) also found subcapsular changes and has shown that pretreatment with pilocarpine protected against such changes.

MODE OF ACTION OF IRREVERSIBLE ANTICHOLINESTERASES ON INTRA-OCULAR PRESSURE

In a comparison of the effects of 2 per cent. pilocarpine and 0.03 per cent. or 0.06 percent. echothiophate, Barsam (1972) came to the conclusion that the fall in intra-ocular pressure with echothiophate was the result of an increase in the facility of outflow with no change in aqueous secretion, whereas that with pilocarpine was the result of both increased facility and decreased secretion.

REFERENCES

Abramson, D.H., Franzen, L.A. & Coleman, D.J. Pilocarpine in the presbyope. *Arch. Ophthalmol.*, 89, *100* (1973).
Abramson, D.H., Chang, S., Coleman, D.J. & Smith, M.E. Pilocarpine-induced lens changes. An ultrasonic biometric evaluation of dose response. *Arch. Ophthalmol.*, 92, *464* (1974).
Alm, A., Bill, A. & Young, F.A. The effect of pilocarpine and neostigmine on the

blood flow through the anterior uvea in monkeys. A study with radioactively labelled microspheres. *Exp. Eye Res.*, 15, *31* (1973).

Armaly, M.F. & Rao, K.R. The effect of pilocarpine Ocusert on ocular pressures. In 'Symposium on ocular therapy. Vol. 6'. (I.H. Leopold, editor). The C.V. Mosby Co., St. Louis (1973).

Axelsson, U. & Holmberg, A. The frequency of cataract after miotic therapy. *Acta Ophthalmol.* 44, *421* (1966).

Bárány, E.H. The mode of action of pilocarpine on outflow resistance of the eye of a primate (Cercopithecus ethiops). *Invest. Ophthalmol.*, 1, *712* (1962).

Bárány, E.H. Dissociation of accommodation effects from outflow effects of pilocarpine. In 'Drug Mechanisms in Glaucoma' (G. Paterson, S.J.H. Miller & G.D. Paterson, editors). Churchill, London (1966).

Bárány, E.H. The immediate effect on outflow resistance of intravenous pilocarpine in the vervet monkey (Cercopithecus ethiops). *Invest. Ophthalmol.*, 6, *373* (1967).

Barsam, P.C. Comparison of the effect of 2% pilocarpine and echothiophate on intraocular pressure and outflow facility. *Am. J. Ophthalmol.*, 73, *742* (1972).

Berggren, L. Effect of parasympathomimetic and sympathomimetic drugs on secretion in vitro by the ciliary processes of the rabbit eye. *Invest. Ophthalmol.*, 4, *91* (1965).

Dale, H.H. The action of certain esters and ethers of choline and their relation to muscarine. *J. Pharmac. exp. Ther.*, 6, *147* (1914).

Dannheim, R. & Bárány, E.H. The effect of trabeculotomy in normal eyes of rhesus and cynomolgus monkeys studied by anterior chamber perfusion. *Document. Ophthalmol.* (Den Haag), 26, *90* (1969).

Demailly, P. Place de l'aceclidine dans le traitement du glaucome chronique simple à angle ouvert. *Arch. Ophthal.*, 28, *735* (1968).

Drance, S.M. & Nash, P.A. The dose response of human intra-ocular pressure of pilocarpine. *Can. J. Ophthalmol.*, 6, *9* (1971).

Drance, S.M., Fairclough, M. & Schulzer, M. Dose response curve of human intra-ocular pressure to aceclidine. *Arch. Ophthalmol.*, 88, *394* (1972).

Drance, S.M., Bensted, M. Schulzer, M. Pilocarpine and intra-ocular pressure; duration and effectiveness of 4% and 8% pilocarpine instillation. *Arch. Ophthalmol.*, 91, *104* (1974).

Ellingson, B.A. & Grant, W.M. Influence of intra-ocular pressure and trabeculotomy on aqueous outflow in enucleated monkey eyes. *Invest. Ophthalmol.*, 10, *705* (1971).

Etienne, R., Barut, C. & Gonzales-Bouchon, J. A new ocular hypotensive, aceclydine. *Ann. Oculist.*, 200, *287* (1967).

Fechner, P.U., Teichmann, K.D. & Weyrauch, W. Accommodative effects of aceclidine in the treatment of glaucoma. *Am. J. Ophthalmol.*, 79, *104* (1975).

Glees, M. & Wurstenberg, W. Experiences with Mintacol in the normal and glaucomatous eye. *Klin. Monatsbl. F. Augenh.*, 114, *454* (1949).

Grant, W.M. Further studies on facility of flow through the trabecular meshwork. *Arch. Ophthalmol.*, 60, *523* (1958).

Grant, W.M. Experimental aqueous perfusion in enucleated human eyes. *Arch. Ophthalmol.*, 69, *783* (1963).

Harris, L.S. & Galin, M.A. Dose response analysis of pilocarpine-induced ocular hypotension. *Arch. Ophthalmol.*, 84, *605* (1970).

Harris, L.S. & Galin, M.A. Effect of ocular pigmentation on hypotensive response to pilocarpine. *Am. J. Ophthalmol.*, 72, *923* (1971).

Hobbiger, F. Cholinergic innervation and the effects of parasympathomimetic drugs. In 'Drug Mechanisms in Glaucoma'. (G. Paterson, S.J.H. Miller & G.D. Paterson, editors). Churchill, London (1966).

Holland, M.G. Autonomic drugs in ophthalmology: some problems and promises. *Ann. Ophthalmol.*, 6, *447* (1974).

Koelle, G.B. & Friedenwald, J.S. A histochemical method for localizing cholinesterase activity. *Proc. Soc. Exp. Biol.*, 70, *617* (1949).

Leopold, I.H. Anticholinesterase agents in glaucoma therapy. In 'Drug Mechanisms in Glaucoma'. (G. Paterson, S.J.H. Miller & G.D. Paterson, editors). Churchill, London (1966).

Leopold, I.H. & Comroe, J.H. Use of di-isopropyl fluorophosphate (DFP) in treatment of glaucoma. *Arch. Ophthalmol.*, 36, *1* (1946).

Leopold, I.H., Gold, P. & Gold, D. Use of thiophosphinyl quaternary compound (217 MI) in treatment of glaucoma. *Arch. Ophthalmol.*, 58, *363* (1957).

Levene, R.Z. Echothiophate iodide and lens changes. In 'Symposium on Ocular Therapy. Volume 4' (I.H. Leopold, editor). The C.V. Mosby Co., St. Louis (1969).

Liebermann, T.W. & Leopold, I.H. The use of aceclydine in the treatment of glaucoma: its effect on intra-ocular pressure and facility of aqueous humour outflow as compared to that of pilocarpine. *Am. J. Ophthalmol.* 64, *405* (1967).

Lyons, J.S. & Krohn, D.L. Pilocarpine uptake by pigmented uveal tissue. *Am. J. Ophthalmol.*, 75, *885* (1973).

O'Brien, C.S. & Swan, K.C. Carbaminoylcholine chloride in the treatment of glaucoma simplex. *Arch. Ophthalmol.*, 27, *253* (1942).

Peterson, W.S., Jocson, V.L. & Sears, M.L. Resistance to aqueous outflow in the rhesus monkey eye. *Am. J. Ophthalmol.* 72, *445* (1971).

de Robertis, E. 'Synaptic receptors: isolation and molecular biology'. Marcel Dekker, New York (1975).

de Roetth, A., Jr. Lens opacities in glaucoma patients on Phospholine Iodide therapy. *Am. J. Ophthalmol.*, 62, *619* (1966).

Romano, J.H. Double-blind cross-over comparison of aceclidine and pilocarpine in open-angle glaucoma. *Acta Ophthalmol.*, 54, *510* (1970).

Shaffer, R.N. & Hetherington, J., Jr. Anticholinesterases and cataracts. *Am. J. Ophthalmol.*, 62, *613* (1966).

Tarkkanen, A. & Karjalainen, K. Cataract formation during miotic therapy for chronic open-angle glaucoma. *Acta Ophthalmol.*, 44, *932* (1966).

Törnqvist, G. Comparative studies of the effect of pilocarpine on the pupil and on the refraction in two species of monkey, (Cercopithecus ethiops and Macaca irus). *Invest. Ophthalmol.*, 3, *388* (1964).

Törnqvist, G. Accommodation in monkeys. *Acta Ophthalmol.*, 45, *429* (1967).

Tripathi, R.C. Ultrastructure of Schlemm's canal in relation to aqueous outflow. *Exp. Eye Res.*, 1, *335* (1968).

Tripathi, R.C. Aqueous outflow pathway in normal and glaucomatous eyes. *Br. J. Ophthalmol.*, 56, *157* (1972).

Tripathi, R.C. Comparative physiology and anatomy of the outflow pathway. In: 'The Eye. Volume 5. Comparative Physiology.' (H. Davson & L.T. Graham, Jr., editors). Academic Press, London (1974).

Uusitalo, R. & Palkama, A. Evidence for the nervous control of secretion in the ciliary processes. *Prog. Brain Res.*, 34, *513* (1972).

Uusitalo, R., Stjernschantz, J. & Palkama, A. Studies on parasympathetic control of the blood-aqueous barrier in the rabbit. An electron microscopic study. *Exp. Eye Res.*, 19, *125* (1974).

Weber, A. Quoted by Goodman, L.S. & Gilman, A. 'The Pharmacological Basis of Therapeutics' 2nd Edn. p. 470. New York, Macmillan (1955).

Author's address:
c/o Moorfield Hospital
High Holborn
London WC 1 V7AN
England

CHOLINERGIC DRUGS: DIRECT PARASYMPATHOMIMETIC DRUGS

E.L. GREVE

(Amsterdam)

Miotic therapy is still one of the pillars of medical therapy in glaucoma. The drugs are known to all of you and are probably used by all of you. The new developments of miotic therapy are not in the drugs themselves but in the way of administration of the drug. It is however useful to evaluate what we are doing with miotic therapy and to realize that miotic therapy is not without problems.

Miotic therapy is the oldest non-surgical therapy of glaucoma and we celebrate today the 100 year anniversary of Pilocarpine and Eserine. It was in 1876 that Laqueur discovered Eserine and that Weber discovered Pilocarpine.

The parasympathomimetic drugs can be subdivided in direct and indirect action. I shall discuss the direct parasympathomimetic drugs and Dr Dake will discuss the indirect parasympathomimetic drugs.

MODE OF ACTION

The action of cholinergic drugs in the eye is mainly on the ciliary muscles, on the constrictor muscle of the pupil, and on the levator muscle. They also cause vasodilitation. For chronic simple glaucoma the action on the ciliary body is the most important (fig. 1). The long ciliary muscle attaches to the sceral spur and by contraction opens the trabecular meshwork. A second action of the ciliary muscles is the release of tension of the zonulae lentis which results in accomodation. The third action is that the plane of lens-ciliary body moves forward which results in narrowing of the anterior chamber (fig. 2). The pressure lowering effect due to action on the ciliar muscle is accompagnied by a miotic effect due to contraction of the constrictor muscle of the pupil. The effect of the outflow and on the pupil are not linked. The increase of outflow after for instance pilocarpine remains present if pilocarpine is combined with a mydriatic drug. If the long ciliary muscle is cut off at the insertion at the scleral spur so that it can not exert its action on the trabecular meshwork, a drop of pilocarpine does not produce any pressure lowering effect although it does produce a miosis. This illustrates clearly that the pressure lowering effect and the miotic effect of cholinergic drugs is dissociated. The amount of miosis is not a control for the pressure lowering effect of cholinergic drugs. Miosis is not essential for medical therapy in chronic simple wide angle glaucoma. On the other hand for angle closure glaucoma the effect on the pupil is essential. Here the effect on the ciliary muscle is a side effect that is not entirely desirable in all cases. This difference in action of cholinergic drugs for chronic simple glaucoma and for angle closure glaucoma should be kept in mind.

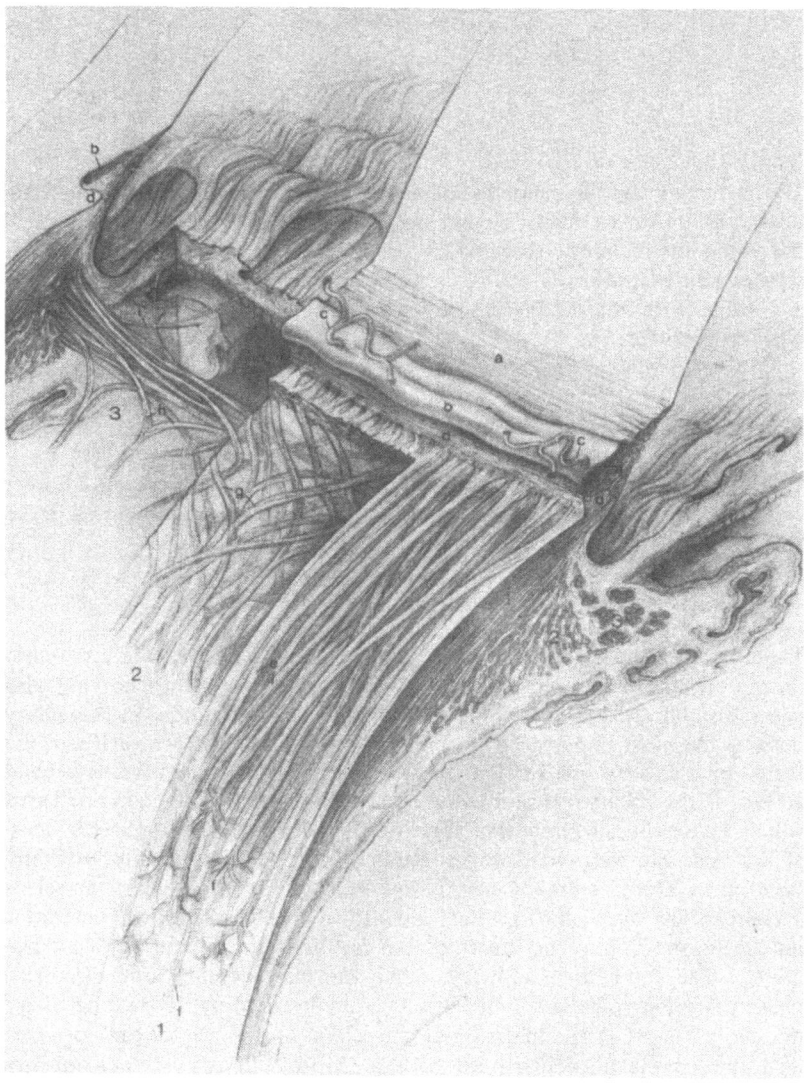

Fig. 1 Anatomy of the ciliary muscle (after Hogan *et al.* 1971). 1. Longitudinal ciliary muscle; 2. radical ciliary muscle; 3. circular ciliary muscle; a. trabecular meshwork; b. Schlemm's canal; c. collector channels; d. scleral spur.

The direct parasympathomimetic drugs are short acting drugs. Stimulated by desire to find longer acting drugs, the cholinesterase inhibitors have been found. As we will see the side effects of most of these longer acting drugs are such that they are hardly used in the uncomplicated simple glaucoma case. This means that we have to rely on the short acting direct parasympathomimetic drugs. The duration of the short acting drug is usually 4 to 6 hours. Shorter intervals between administration of eye drops is not acceptable to the patient unless there is an emergency. The usual 6 hour regime results in a pulsed dosage (fig. 3). An overdose alternates with an underdose. During the overdose stage one can expect side effects like for instance miosis and accomodation. During the underdose stage one may wonder whether the drug still exerts its effect on IOP. This pulsed dosage regime is a specific problem of short acting miotics like pilocarpine. A second problem that is inherent to short-acting miotics is that it is difficult to control the IOP during the night. An action of 4 hours is not sufficient for the usual sleeping period of 8 hours.

SIDE EFFECTS

The side effects of the cholinergic drugs can be subdivided in local and general side effects. The local side effects are very frequent while the general side effects are extremely rare.

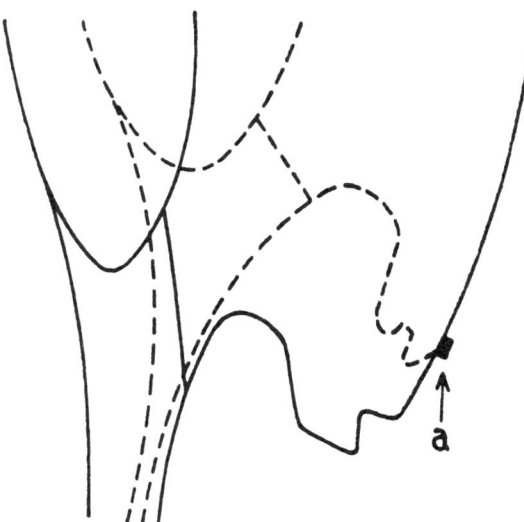

Fig. 2. Effect of atropine and eserine on the position of the iris-lens-ciliary body position (from Duke-Elder, 1961). The continuous line shows the position of the ciliary body and lens under the influence of atropine; the broken line under the influence of eserine. a. indicates the position of the scleral spur.

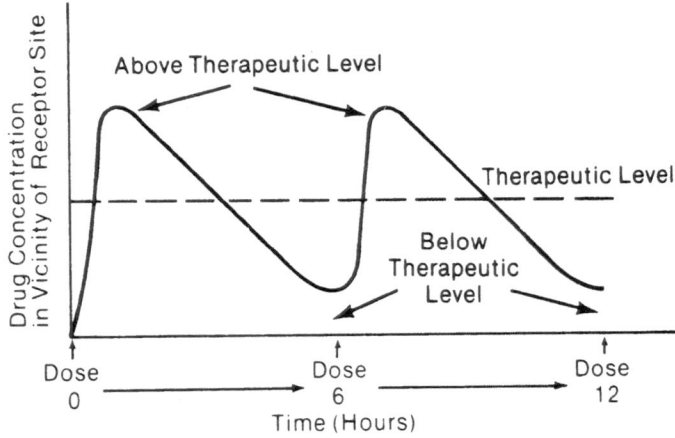

Fig. 3. The pulsed dosage effect of short-acting cholinergic drugs.

LOCAL SIDE EFFECTS

Ciliary spasm causes pain in the form of a browe-ache that usually de-minishes after some days of use of the drug. For some people however this pain remains intolerable. The worst side effect caused by ciliary spasm specially in young people is the induced myopia. This myopia can be as much as 8 diopters and is larger in myopes than in emmetropes or hyper-metropes. In combination with miosis the myopia may give visual distur-bances that are un-acceptable for certain professions. Ciliary spasm has also been blamed for the occurrence of the retinal detachments after cholinergic drugs. The shallowing of the anterior chamber that accompanies the use of cholinergic drugs can have a dangerous effect in angle closure glaucoma. Where the aim of miotic therapy in angle closure glaucoma is to free the trabecular meshwork from the iris-base, the anterior chamber shallowing effect of the drug by a forward movement of the ciliary body may have an antagonistic action on the IOP.

Miosis is also one of the undesired side effects of miotic therapy. After installation of the miotic drops the patient experiences a period of semi-darkness. Specially at night a bad vision may result from the miotic which presents serious driving problems. If a cataract is present the miosis may produce an inacceptable decrease of vision. The use of phenyleprine 5% may counteract the miotic effect in wide angle glaucoma.

A second effect of the miosis may be a pupillary block. Together with the forward displacement of the ciliary body, the pupillary block may counteract the action that frees trabecular meshwork from the iris base.

It is well known that after a long term use of miotics the sphincter may become very rigid. It may be difficult to dilate the pupil in such patients and because of the lack of dillatation it may be impossible to get a good stereo-scopic view of the optic disc. The sphincter rigidity may also be an obstacle in cataract extraction.

The vascular congestion often causes a red eye. It sometimes causes aqueous flare, posterior synechiae and iris cysts. These last three side effects are rarely seen after the use of direct parasympathomimetic drugs. Tearing is a frequent but not so important complain after miotic therapy. Twitching of the eyelid is not so frequent. Like with all other drugs an allergic or toxic reactions may occur.

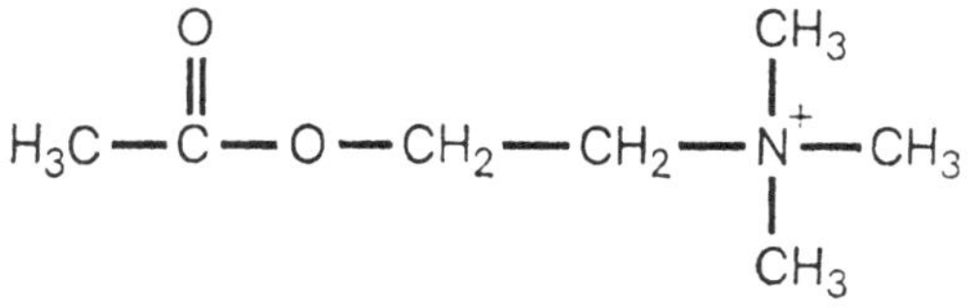

$$H_3C-\overset{\overset{\displaystyle O}{\|}}{C}-O-CH_2-CH_2-\overset{\overset{\displaystyle CH_3}{|}}{\underset{\underset{\displaystyle CH_3}{|}}{N^+}}-CH_3$$

Fig. 4. Structure of acetyl-choline.

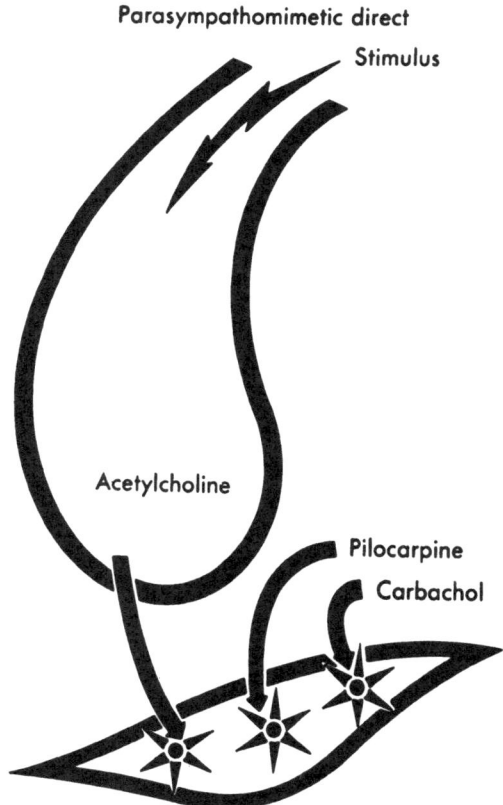

Fig. 5. Action of acetyl-choline, pilocarpine and carbachol (after Richardson, 1970). Acetyl-choline is manufactured and stored within the parasympathetic neuron. It stimulates the effect or cell directly. Pilocarpine and carbachol mimick this action.

It has recently been described that pilocarpine has a cataractogenous effect. In a follow-up study of 30 patients that were treated in one eye with pilocarpine, six treated eyes showed more lens opacities after a five year period than the untreated eyes. The frequency and extent of these lens opacities is much less than that caused by cholinesterase inhibitors lit,...).

Adaptation to cholinergic drugs may always occur. If it happens and is detected it is useful to stop the particular drug and alternate with an other cholinergic drug. After some time the original sensitivity to the first drug will come back.

GENERAL SIDE EFFECTS

General side effects of cholinergic drugs are very rare but have been described in cases who were treated for angle closure glaucoma. The symptoms are transpiration, weakness, feeling of illness, vivid dreams, depressions and delusions. Gastro-intestinal symptoms include saliorrhoea, stomach pain, diarrhoea etc. Pulmonary symptoms are those of increased secretion, bronchoconstriction and asthma bronchinale. Cardiac symptoms are bradycardia, heard standstill, arythmias and collaps. Parasthesias may occur.

CHOLINERGIC DRUGS

Acetylcholine

Acetylcholine is the physiological mediator of the parasympathic response (fig. 4). It stimulates directly the endplate where it interacts with the celmembrane which causes depolarization (fig. 5). Acetylcholine is rapidly broken down by cholinesterase. It has a very low corneal permeability. Its application is limited to use intra-camera during operations.

Metacholine

Methacholine is very similar to acetylcholine. It is also short acting and has a low corneal permeability. It has no application in glaucoma.

Pilocarpine

Pilocarpine has been used for the best part of hundred years. It is usually the first drug prescribed for a raised IOP. Its possibilities will probably be even wider now that it is available in membranes for sustained release. Pilocarpine is an alkaloid of pilocarpus jaborandi (fig. 6). Its action is direct on the muscle. Pilocarpine exists in equilibrium between undissociated lipid soluble and it is dissociated water soluble form. It penetrates the corneal epithelium in water soluble form and works better in a basic milieu. It is available as nitrate, as hydrochloride, in methylcellulose, in oil, in ointment, in soft lenses, and in ocusert.

Pilocarpine produces a miosis after 10 to 15 minutes which lasts 4 to 8 hours. It has been said already the miosis is not equivalent to IOP reduction. The effect on IOP is maximal after two hours as can be seen in figure 7. The maximum reduction of IOP and the duration of this effect depends on the concentration of pilocarpine and the pigmentation of the iris (see table 1). The average reduction of IOP is 25%. It may vary from 12 to 40% (fig. 8). The duration of action on average is 4 to 6 hours, but there is a large inter-individual variation. The pressure lowering effect of 8% pilo-

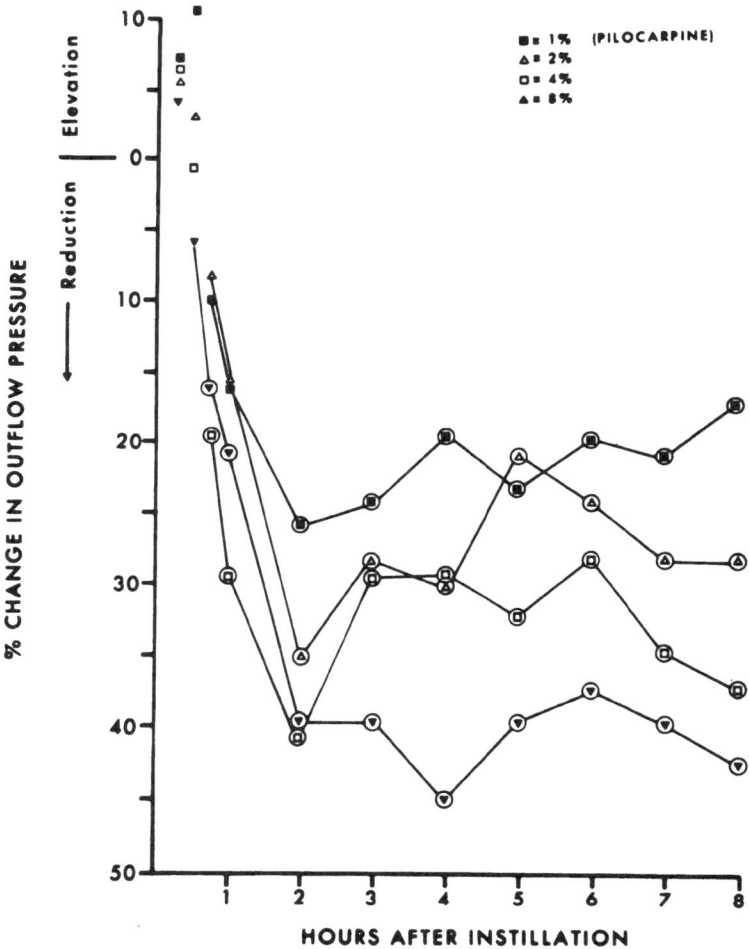

Fig. 6   Structure of pilocarpine.

Fig. 7. Pressure reducing effect of different concentrations of pilocarpine. (after Drance & Nash; 1971).

31

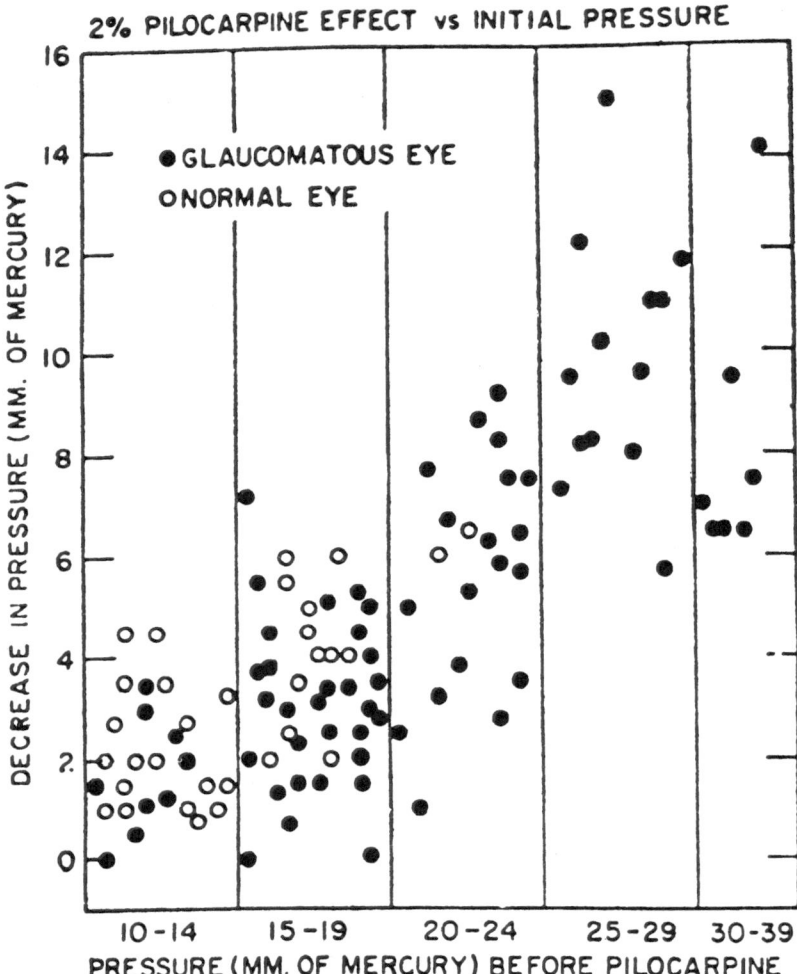

Fig. 8. Effect of pilocarpine 2% on IOP. The absolute effect depends on the level of the initial IOP-level. The percentage effect is approximately the same for all IOP levels (after Krill & Newell; 1964)

carpine is usually not more than that of 4% pilocarpine but its duration is longer. The duration can be up to 8 hours which might be of importance for controlling the IOP during the night. A second effect of cholinergic drugs is that the diurnal variation usually diminishes. From the above mentioned facts it is clear that pilocarpine drops should be tested in different concentrations for different individuals. One should not stick to the use of 2% pilocarpine.

The side effects of pilocarpine are those mentioned under the general heading of cholinergic drugs. The problems are mainly caused by the pulsed dosage. As we will see some of these problems have been overcome by the use of ocusert.

Aceclidine is a synthetic drug that was recently developed in Russia (fig. 9). It is the second choice in miotic therapy and sometimes the first choice. Its action is like pilocarpine direct on the muscle. In our country the available glaucostat is aceclidine-hydrochloride. It penetrates the cornea well. The effect on the IOP of 2% aceclidine is approximately the same as that of pilocarpine 2% (Table 2). Aceclidine is well tolerated. It is said that it produces less myopia than pilocarpine but this is not our clinical experience. For this reason some doctors begin with aceclidine instead of pilocarpine in young patients. Another advantage of aceclidine is its unlimited conservation in dry form. In solution it can be used for approximately four weeks.

TABLE 1. Effect of pilocarpine on IOP related to colour of the iris (after Harris & Galin; 1971)

Percentage IOP reduction

iriscolour	1%	4%	8%
caucasian blue	30.0	34.8	36.0
caucasian brown	15.3	26.1	28.0
black brown	13.8	18.5	22.2

TABLE 2. Comparison of the effect on IOP of different concentrations of pilocarpine and carbachol.

Pilocarpine	Carbachol	Aceclidine
1	0.75	–
2	1.50	2
4	2.25	–
8	3.00	–

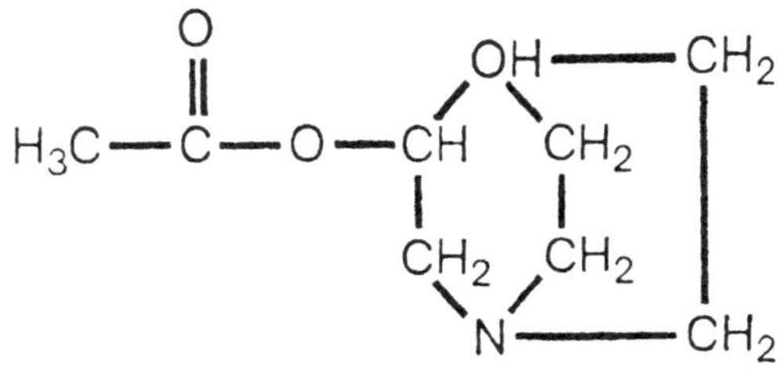

Fig. 9. Structure of aceclidine.

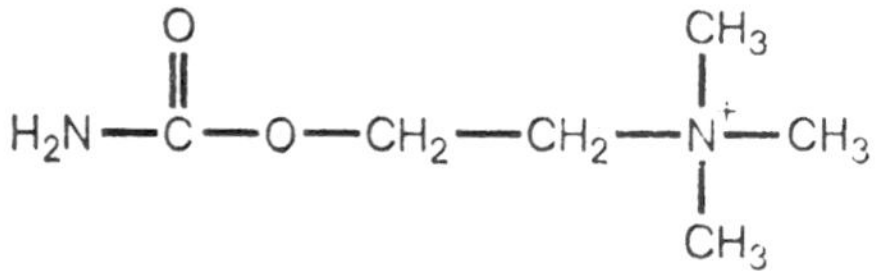

Fig. 10. Structure of carbachol.

Aceclidine has been combined with epinephrine in one eye drop which offers an easy administration for the patient. The combined drops, glaucodrine, can be prescribed twice a day in combination with twice a day glaucostat so that the patient receives in total four administrations per day. This form of treatment seems to be equivalent with the combination of pilocarpine and epinephrine drops separately.

Carbachol

Carbachol is also a synthetic drug and differs only slightly from acetylcholine (fig. 10). Its breakdown by cholinesterase is slower than that of acetylcholine so that the drug can be used in glaucoma. Its action is mainly direct on the muscle but there is also an inhibiting action on acetylcholinesterase. Carbachol has a bad lipid solubility and does not penetrate the corneal epithelium unless it is used in methylcellulose. In our country it is available in methylcellulose 1% as isoptocarbachol in a concentration of 1.5 and 3.0%. The effect of 1.5% carbachol on IOP is comparable with that of pilocarpine 2% (Table 2). The duration of the pressure reduction of 3% carbachol is approximately 8 hours and comparable with that of 8% pilocarpine. The miosis lasts three times longer than that of pilocarpine. The side effects are a little stronger than those of pilocarpine. Headaches are more pronounced and the vasodilatation effect is stronger. Like in pilocarpine it is important to test the different percentages of carbachol in the individual. Carbachol is a good alternative for pilocarpine specially if adaptation to pilocarpine occurs or if the patient is hypersensitive to pilocarpine.

These three drugs are the direct parasympathomimetic drugs that are used at present. Do not say too quickly that the direct cholinergic drugs do not work. Try several concentrations and/or vehicles.

REFERENCES AND RECOMMENDED LITERATURE

Drance, S.M. & Nash, P.A. The dose responce of human intra-ocular pressure to pilocarpine. *Canad. J. Ophthal.* 6 : 9 (1971).

Drance, S.M. Use of cholinergic agents in the management of chronic simple glaucoma. Trans. New. Orleans. Acad. Ophthal. Mosby, St Louis. p. 32. (1970).

Duke-Elder, S. & Wybar, K.C. System of Ophthalmology vol II. H. Kimpton London; (1961).

Havener, W.H. Ocular pharmacology. Mosby St. Louis. 1974.

Harris, L.S. & Galin, M.A. Pilocarpine response and eye color. *Amer. J. Ophthal.* 72 : 376, (1975)

Hogan, M.J., Alverado, J.A. & Esperson, J. Histology of the human eye. W.B. Saunders Co. Philadephia (1971).

Krill, A., Newell, F. Effects of pilocarpine on ocular tension dynamics. *Amer. J. Ophthal. 57 : 34*, (1964).

Levene, R.Z. Uniocular miotic therapy. *Trans. Amer. Acad. Ophthal. 79, 376* (1975).

Richardson, K. Autonomic pharmacology. Trans. New Orleans. Acad. Ophthal. Mosby, St. Louis, p. 32. 1970.

Author's address:
Eye Clinic of the University of Amsterdam
Wilhelmina Gasthuis
Eerste Helmerstraat 104
Amsterdam
The Netherlands

INDIRECT PARASYMPATHOMIMETIC DRUGS

C.L. DAKE

(Amsterdam)

I shall give a short clinical survey about anticholinesterase drugs. They act by inhibition of cholinesterase. Through inhibition of this enzyme hydrolyzation of acethylcholine is prevented and all cholinergic effects are produced by sensitizing the receptor mechanism to parasympathetic stimulation. Like cholinergic drugs cholinesterase inhibitors produce an increase of facility of outflow.

This survey will be limited to drugs that are obtainable in Holland.

Anticholinesterase drugs can be divided into **carbonates** and **organophosphates**.

To the **carbonates** belong Eserine or Physostigmine, a naturally occurring alkaloid, and Demecariumbromide, a synthetic product.

Eserine is the oldest antiglaucomatous drug and was used for the first time in 1876 by Laqueur. It inhibits the action of acethylcholinesterase by forming a reversible compound with the enzyme. This results in a gradual return of enzymatic activity when the inhibited enzyme is exposed to acethylcholine. Eserine is used as the salicylate in solutions of 0.25% to 1%. The parasympathetic action is stronger than that of pilocarpine, giving an intense miosis and ciliary spasm. Prolonged use frequently results in an allergic irritation of the conjunctiva and sometimes the formation of cysts at the pupillary margin is seen.

Although eserine is often combined with pilocarpine, so-called 'Misch-Tropfen', the investigations of Kronfeld (1967), cast some doubt upon the efficacy of this prescription; there is evidence that such a combination has no greater effect than its most potent component.

The popularity of eserine has waned in recent years, probably because it is not very stable in solution, and because of its side effects.

Demecariumbromide (syn. Humorsol and Tosmilen) is obtainable in Holland in a 0,25% concentration. It forms a much more stable, though still reversible, inhibited enzyme. Its action is comparable to the organophosphates and it has the same side effects. It is water soluble and stable at room temperature. Because of its long action the use should be limited to once or twice a day and sometimes even less.

We do not have experience of any importance with this drug.

To the **organophosphates** belong Mintacol and Echothiophate. They react with cholinesterase to form a phosphorylated enzyme; such an enzyme

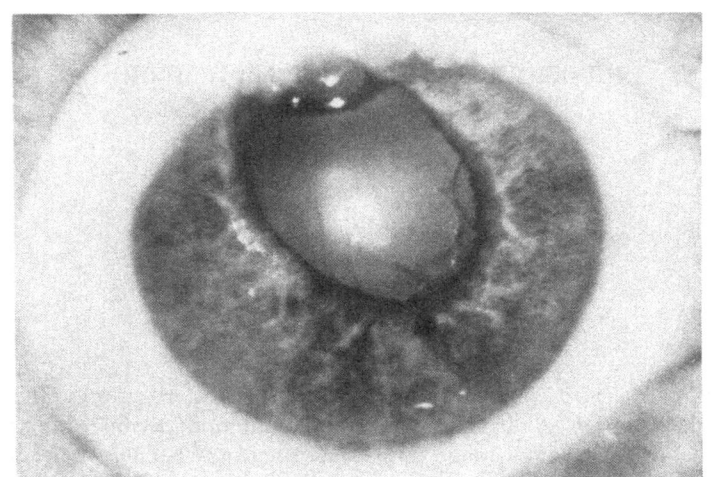

Fig. 1. R. eye. pat. 1.

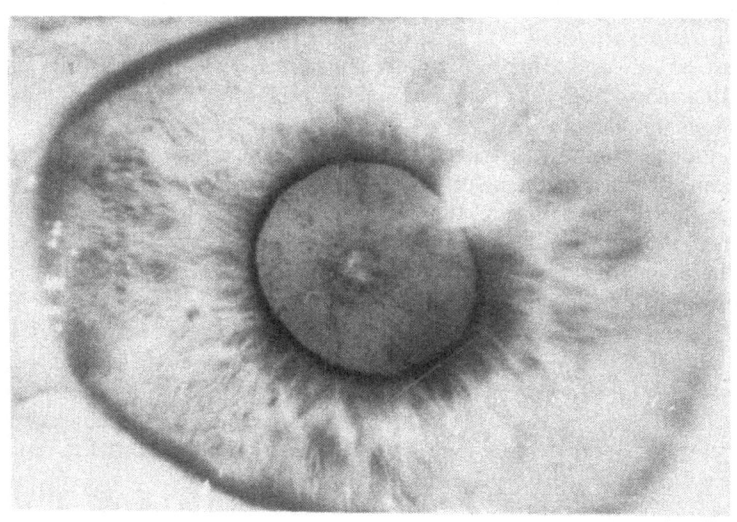

Fig. 2. L. eye. pat. 1.

shows only a very slow spontaneous reactiviation. Therefore they are called 'irreversible' inhibitors.

Mintacol or di-ethyl-p-nitrophenylphosphate is used in 0,25% to 1% solutions. Since the advent of epinephrine and carbonic anhydrase inhibitors its use has been declining. Publications on accelerated cataract formation have given a further decrease in its use. Although quite frequently used in Amsterdam in the past we have not been aware of this cataractogenic effect.

Echothiophate or Phospholine Iodide is water soluble and stable at 4° C. It can be kept in solution for at least six months at this temperature, at room temperature only 30 days. Concentrations vary between 0,03% and 0,250%.

Side effects: Anticholinesterase drugs and in particular Tosmilen and the organophosphates produce local and systemic side effects. The local effects include ocular pain and frontal headache due to ciliary spasm, intense miosis that can last several weeks, myopia, pigment dispersion in the anterior chamber, posterior synechia, pigment cysts at the pupillary margin and sometimes anterior uveitis.

Pupillary block is increased and the depth of the anterior chamber decreased; through this mechanism an attack of angle closure glaucoma can be precipitated in eyes with a narrow angle.

Retinal detachment can be induced through traction at the ciliary body.

The frequent occurrence of lens opacities (40-80%) has been stressed by Axelsson, Holmberg (1966), de Roeth (1966), Shaffer and Hetherington (1966). From 17 patients in our hospital who used Phospholine Iodide between 8 and 24 months 10 developed a cataract. Nine of them were sixty years or over, one was 50 years old (Dake 1968). The 0,03% Phospholine Iodide solution has not yet shown to be cataractogenic, but its action on IOP is not better than that of pilocarpine 1% or 2%.

The following figures of 2 patients are instructive. Fig. 1 shows the R eye of a 68-year-old man, operated in June 1965. The eye got Phospholine Iodide drops. Both eyes had a visual acuity of 5/5. After ten months vision in the L eye was 5/10 and 5 months later had dropped to 5/50. Vision in the R eye was still 5/5. Fig. 2 shows the cataract in the L eye. The second patient was 74 years old and the visual acuity of the R eye was 5/10, L eye 5/20. The R eye was operated twice in 1965; first a peripheral iridencleisis, and, because of insufficient pressure reduction, followed by a sector iridencleises 3 months later. The L eye received phospholine iodide during 15 months. After that period the visual acuity of the R eye was 5/15 and of the L eye only H.M. (fig. 3 and 4).

Topical use of phospholine iodide can result in enough systemic absorption to decrease the cholinesterase content in erythrocytes and serum. This can cause systemic side effects like abdominal dyscomfort, diarrhoea, vomiting, bradycardia, systemic hypotension and muscular weakness.

If succinylcholine is used in general anaesthesia this can cause prolonged respiratory arrest because succinylcholine is broken down by cholinesterase.

Our conclusion is that irreversible cholinesterase inhibitors are strong miotic drugs, but they have many side effects. Some of them are so serious, particularly in the phakic patient, that we recommend it only in glaucoma

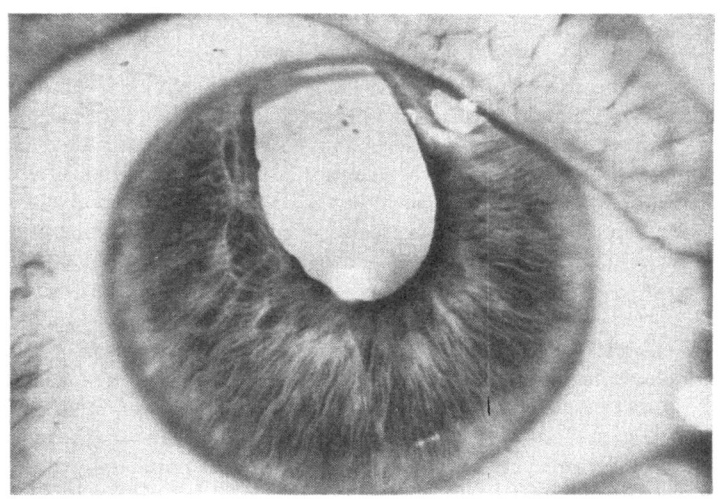

Fig. 3. R. eye. pat. II.

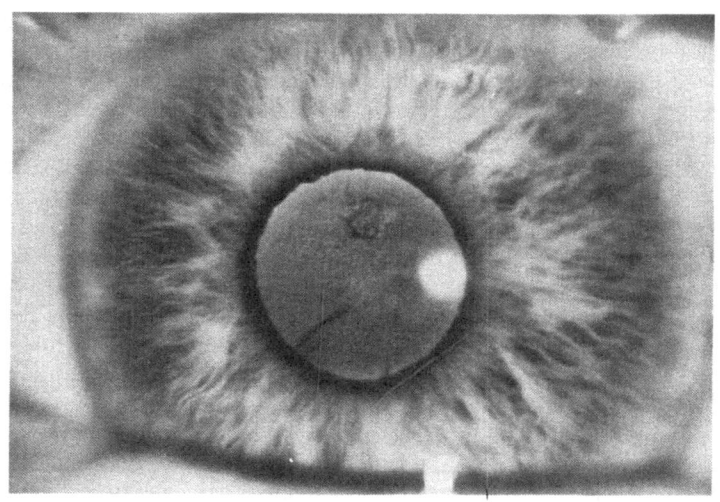

Fig. 4. L. eye. pat. II.

40

with aphakia, provided that there is no history or sign of predisposition to retinal detachment. They are contra-indicated in chronic glaucoma with a narrow angle.

REFERENCES

Axelsson, U., Holmberg, A. The frequency of cataract after miotic therapy. *Acta Ophthal. (kbh)* 44, *421-429* (1966).

Dake, C.L., Kerlen, C.H. Fosfoline iodide en lenstroebeling. *Ned. T. Geneesk.* 112, *1898-1901* (1968).

Kronfeld, P.C. The efficacy of combinations of ocular hypotensive drugs. *Arch. Ophthal.* 78, *140-146* (1967).

Roetth, A. de. Lens opacities in glaucoma patients on phospholine iodide therapy. *Amer. J. Ophthal.* 62, *613-618* (1966).

Shaffer, R.N., Hetherington, Jr., J. Anticholinesterase drugs and cataracts. *Amer. J. Ophthal.* 62, *613-618* (1966).

Author's address:
Eye Clinic of the University of Amsterdam
Wilhelmina Gasthuis
Eerste Helmerstraat 104
Amsterdam
The Netherlands

EXPERIENCES WITH OCUSERT

F.E. ROS, E.L. GREVE, C.L. DAKE & W.M. MILLER

(Amsterdam)

Introduction

The Ocusert pilocarpine system is the first membrane-controlled drug delivery system with clinical acceptance in ophthalmology. Richardson (1975) gave us an excellent review of membrane-controlled drug delivery in ophthalmology. For the reader we give here a short abstract from Richardson's papers, because it is necessary for the understanding of the working mechanism of Ocusert and its place among other systems. The articles of Richardson are highly recommended.

As Richardson states 'membrane-controlled drug-delivery systems are a platform for design of optimal therapeutic regimens and, if they achieve their promise, an exciting even revolutionary concept in therapy with virtually unlimited horizons'.

Until now physicians struggled with the fact that, with the exception of continuous intravenous therapy, a constant and continuous administration of a drug was impossible. Conventional dosage forms, like eye-drops, give a periodic rise and fall in body fluid levels of the drug. The conventional alternating overdose-underdose delivery of drugs is known as first-order drug delivery rate. A substantial disadvantage of this type of regimen is that during the overdose-period more drug is administered than necessary to achieve the therapeutic goal, which entails a higher possibility of side effects.

From a standpoint of practical clinical therapeutics the most useful pharmaco-kinetic relationship is that, which is obtained with a constant rate of drug delivery. This has been known as zero-order drug delivery rate. It can be achieved by newly designed drug delivery systems.

Synthetic polymeric membranes play an important role in the efforts to produce a controlled drug delivery system. Functionally the most important property of a synthetic polymeric membrane is its permeability. Furthermore, the fact that the characteristics of a given membrane have to be compatible with whose of a given drug, cannot be overemphasized.

For zero-order drug delivery non porous membranes are used. Synthetic polymeric membranes have been used in a variety of forms:

1. **Prolonged or sustained delivery** (but still first order).

a) Drug dissolved in membrane (e.g. a soft contactlens soaked in an appropriate solution containing drugs like pilocarpine; more than half of the pilocarpine is released in the first 30 minutes).

b) Drug dispersed in membrane (when a drug is dispersed as a solid in the membrane, the release rate declines much less rapidly than when the drug is dissolved in the membrane).

2. **Controlled delivery** (substantial zero-order delivery).

a) Reservoir module (fig. A). At present the only system available is the Ocusert system, consisting of a central thin film of pilocarpine surrounded by two synthetic copolymeric membranes and a white ring to recognize the

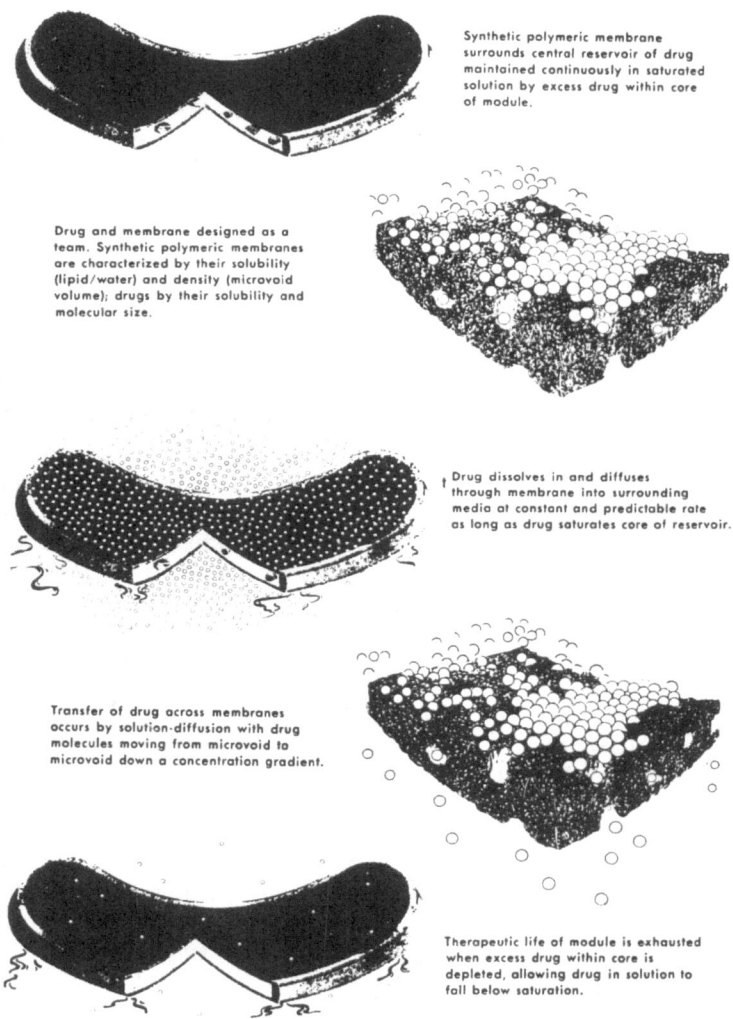

Synthetic polymeric membrane surrounds central reservoir of drug maintained continuously in saturated solution by excess drug within core of module.

Drug and membrane designed as a team. Synthetic polymeric membranes are characterized by their solubility (lipid/water) and density (microvoid volume); drugs by their solubility and molecular size.

Drug dissolves in and diffuses through membrane into surrounding media at constant and predictable rate as long as drug saturates core of reservoir.

Transfer of drug across membranes occurs by solution-diffusion with drug molecules moving from microvoid to microvoid down a concentration gradient.

Therapeutic life of module is exhausted when excess drug within core is depleted, allowing drug in solution to fall below saturation.

Fig. A. Reservoir module for membrane-controlled drug delivery. (After Richardson, K.T., Jr., Membrane-controlled drug delivery. In: The New Orleans Academy of Ophthalmology, Symposium on Glaucoma, 1975. The C.V. Mosby Co., St. Louis, Mo., USA).

44

system. Pilocarpine exists in equilibrium between a water soluble ionized form and a lipid-soluble un-ionized form. The lipid-soluble molecules diffuse from the module when placed in an aqueous medium like the conjunctival sac.

Shortly after manufacture, a small amount of pilocarpine diffuses from the core into the surrounding membrane saturating the membrane with

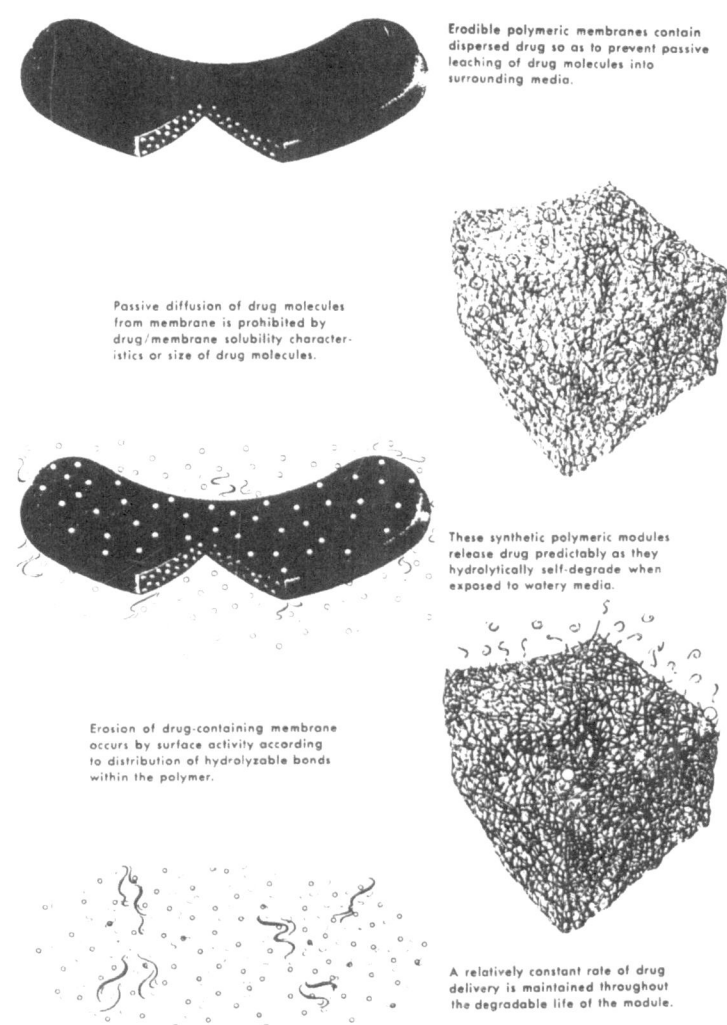

Erodible polymeric membranes contain dispersed drug so as to prevent passive leaching of drug molecules into surrounding media.

Passive diffusion of drug molecules from membrane is prohibited by drug/membrane solubility character-istics or size of drug molecules.

These synthetic polymeric modules release drug predictably as they hydrolytically self-degrade when exposed to watery media.

Erosion of drug-containing membrane occurs by surface activity according to distribution of hydrolyzable bonds within the polymer.

A relatively constant rate of drug delivery is maintained throughout the degradable life of the module.

Fig. B. Erodible module for membrane-controlled drug delivery. (After Richardson, K.T., Jr., Membrane-controlled drug delivery. In: The New Orleans Academy of Opthalmology, Symposium on Glaucoma, 1975. The C.V. Mosby Co., St. Louis, Mo., USA).

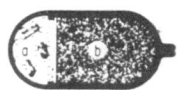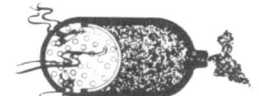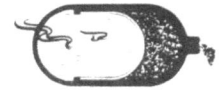

Fig. C. Osmotic module for membrane-controlled drug delivery (After Richardson, K.T., Jr., Membrane-controlled drug delivery. In: The New Orleans Academy of Ophthalmology, Symposium on Glaucoma, 1975. The C.V. Mosby Co., St. Louis, Mo., USA). Drug loaded within the impermeable compartment (*b*) escapes when water from the surrounding media diffuses osmotically into the semipermeable compartment (*a*), causing movement of the elastic intercompartmental membrane. A constant rate of drug delivery occurs as long as excess salt in compartment *a* maintains salt molecules within this compartment in a saturated state.

pilocarpine, and this is responsible for the initial higher release rate when the module is placed in the conjunctival sac. The initial higher release rate exists for approximately 8 hours and reaches then a steady state delivery rate which is constant and continuous during a 7 day period. The constant forces that drive the pilocarpine out of the reservoirs are the blinking, the rapid eye movements and the tear flow.

There are now two Ocusert pilocarpine modules available (see table 7).

b) Erodible module (fig. B). These are synthetic polymeric membranes, that self-degrade during or after the delivery of the drug. The polymer erodes by surface activity usually achieved by a distribution of hydrolyzable bonds within the polymer. When placed in an aqueous medium, the surface polymer molecules are released from the deeper polymers by rupture of the hydrolyzable bonds and the drug contained within the superficial layers of the membrane is simultaneously released.

The advantage of this module could be the less complicated drug/membrane design, because of the somewhat dissimilar solubility characteristics of drug and membrane, in contrast to the reservoir module.

c) Osmotic pumping module (fig. C) (These modules utilize an osmotic pump to deliver drugs at zero-order rate). The drug is loaded within an impermeable compartment, which has a small opening to allow the drug into the surrounding medium. Affixed to this impermeable compartment is a semipermeable container loaded with an appropriate salt, that, when placed in an aqueous medium will imbibe fluid at a zero-order rate as long as the salt is maintained in a saturated state.

Between these two compartments is an elastic membrane, so that when the semipermeable compartments expand the elastic membrane will compromise the impermeable compartment and the drug will be forced through the small opening into the surrounding medium. The advantage of this osmotic pumping system are the less complicated drug membrane design requirements. A possible disadvantage is the relatively smaller flexibility and the size of the system.

Richardson gives an excellent summary of the potential for controlled drug-delivery systems:

46

1. **Zero-order (constant) delivery rate**

a) Avoidance of the overdose/underdose sequence characteristics of intermittent therapy.

b) Reduction in total dosage necessary for disease control.

c) Reduction of systemic absorption in locally treated disease.

d) More effective and reliable prolonged therapy with improved patient compliance.

e) More effective therapy for multicompartmental systems; 1. improvement of drug penetration to slowly accessible areas. 2. improving the therapeutic index when the toxic compartment is different from the therapeutic compartment.

f) Research tool for evaluating; 1. disease responses to different patterns of drug delivery. 2. Defining multicompartmental systems relating to both organs and drugs.

g) Delivery of drugs with poor solubility.

h) Treatment of diseases that respond more appropriately to zero-order-rate drug delivery than to first-order-rate delivery.

2. **Patterned drug delivery rate**

a) Drug delivery patterned to synchronize with or modify biologic rhythms.

b) Therapy of disease when controlled cyclic variation of drug therapy is desirable.

c) Delivery of drugs at a rate triggered by a feedback signal from organ or body.

3. **Multiple sequenced drug therapy**

a) Combinations of drugs, each with a precise, predictable, and different delivery rate.

b) Drug delivery sequencing.

4. **Indirect benefits**

a) Reducing or eliminating the necessity for administration of medication (i.e. postoperative antibiotics, cycloplegics) by inexperienced personnel.

b) Saving of personnel time required by multiple frequent incremental therapy (i.e. postoperative and pre-examination cycloplegic/mydriatics, preoperative antibiotics).

c) Improving therapy in difficult socio-economic environments. (1) Reducing therapeutic failure because of inadequate patient compliance. (2) Reducing therapeutic failure caused by lack of continuously available drug (trachoma). (3) Reducing therapeutic failure of inadequate health personnel patient contact.

In recent years many authors (Armaly & Rao, 1973; Bucci, 1972; Worthen et al., 1974; Friederich, 1974; Heilmann, 1974, 1975; Leydhecker, 1975; Krieglstein, 1975; Drance, 1975; Macoul et al., 1975; Quigley et al., 1975; Place et al., 1975; Lee et al., 1975; Lienert, 1975; Draeger, 1975) reported their clinical experiences with the ocusert-system.

PURPOSE OF OUR STUDY

The purpose of this study was to evaluate the ocular tolerance, patient

TABLE 1. Clinical data of 9 patients with primary glaucoma (established glaucoma 5, glaucoma suspect 4), prestudy medication, current therapy and effect. Abbreviation used are as follows: P1 = Pilocarpine 1% four times daily; P2 = Pilocarpine 2% four times daily; P4 = Pilocarpine 4% four times daily; GS = Glaucostat[R] two times daily; GD = Glaucadrine[R] two times daily; E = Eppy[R] two times daily; I = Isopto Epinal 1% two times daily; AC = Acetazolamide 125 mg three times daily; DFS = Double Flap Scheie; + = significant effect on IOP; no effect P2,P-20 = neither Pilocarpine 2% eye-drops, nor Ocusert P-20 had a significant effect on IOP

ESTABLISHED GLAUCOMA {	wide angle 3	
	narrow angle 2	
	chronic narrow angle –	
(PRIMARY)		
GLAUCOMA SUSPECT {	wide angle 4	
	narrow angle –	
	chronic narrow angle –	

PAT.	AGE	SEX	PRESTUDY MEDICATION		OCUSERT		CONTROL
			OD	OS	OD	OS	ODS
1. F	67	f	P4	P4	P4	P-40	ODS +
2. vR	78	m	P2	P2	P2	P-40	ODS +
3. P	71	m	P2	P2	P-20	P2	ODS +
4. C	74	m	P2	P2 AC	P-20	P2 AC	ODS +
5. B	62	m	P1	P1	P-20	P1	ODS +
6. R	71	f	P2	P2	P-40	P2	ODS +
7. vdW	67	f	P2	P2	P-20	P2	ODS +
8. Z	61	m	P2	P2	P-40,I	P-40,I	ODS +
9. J	55	m	GS	GS AC	P-40	P-20 AC	ODS +

TABLE 2. Clinical data of 1 patient with pigmentary glaucoma, prestudy medication, current therapy and effect. For abbreviations used see table 1.

PAT.	AGE	SEX	PRESTUDY MEDICATION		OCUSERT		CONTROL
			OD	OS	OD	OS	ODS
10. B	41	m	GS,GD	GS,GD	P-20,I	GS,GD	ODS +

compliance and the ocular hypotensive effect of the Ocusert P-20 and P-40 system and to compare this with conventional eyedrop therapy. This comparison was made possible by the use of Ocusert in one eye and eyedrops in the fellow eye.

Patients and methods

We used two different protocols:

Protocol 1: 10 patients treated with Ocusert in one eye or in combination with epinephrine and pilocarpine eyedrops with the same added drug in the fellow eye; this enabled us to compare the long term effect of Ocusert and pilocarpine eye-drop medication, which has not been reported in literature before.

Protocol 2: 11 patients treated with Ocusert in both eyes or patients after filtrating operation with Ocusert in the operated eye or fellow eye.

The initial examination included: visual acuity, slitlamp examination, ophthalmoscopy, applanation tonometry, gonioscopy and visual fields.

The investigation was carried out in 4 phases:

Phase 1: Current therapy was discontinued to obtain two baseline IOP 'diurnal-curves' without therapy. Applanation tonometry was performed at 9,

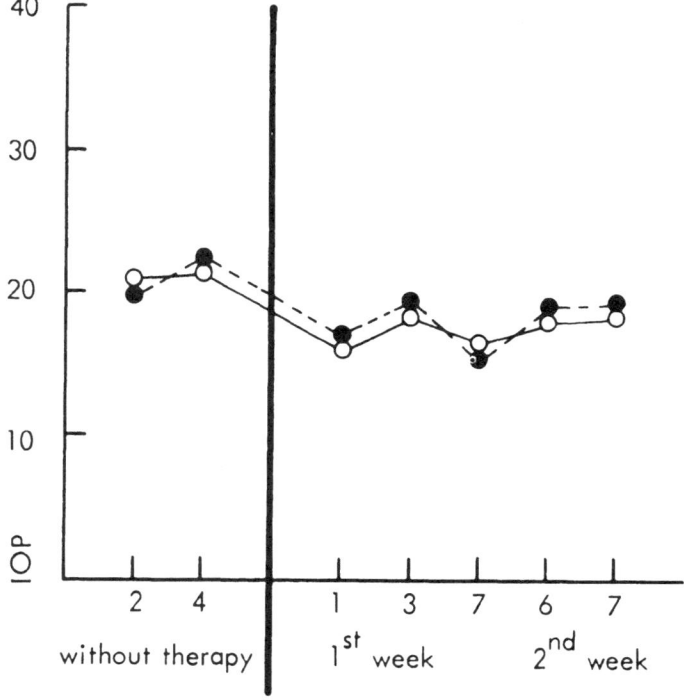

Fig. 1. Patient no. 1; average IOP 2 and 4 days after cessation of therapy. One eye treated with Ocusert P-40 (o), fellow eye with pilocarpine 4% eye-drops four times daily (•).

TABLE 3. Clinical data of 1 patient with low tension glaucoma, prestudy medication, current therapy and effect. For abbreviations used see table 1

PAT.	AGE	SEX	PRESTUDY MEDICATION		OCUSERT		CONTROL
			OD	OS	OD	OS	ODS
11. E	74	f	P2	P2	P2	P-20	no effect P2, P-20

TABLE 4. Clinical data of 1 patient with secondary glaucoma, prestudy medication, current therapy and effect. For abbreviations used see table 1

PAT.	AGE	SEX	PRESTUDY MEDICATION		OCUSERT		CONTROL
			OD	OS	OD	OS	ODS
12. vdW	59	m	GS,GD	GS,GD	GS,GD	P-40,I	ODS +

TABLE 5. Clinical data of 5 patients with primary established glaucoma, prestudy medication, current therapy and result. For abbreviations used see table 1

PRIMARY (ESTABLISHED) GLAUCOMA
{ wide angle 5
  narrow angle –
  chronic narrow angle –

ONE EYE OPERATED, OCUSERT IN THE FELLOW EYE

PAT.	AGE	SEX	PRESTUDY MEDICATION		OCUSERT		CONTROL
			OD	OS	OD	OS	ODS
13. P	64	m	DFS (74)	GS,GD	--- AC	P-40,I	OS no effect GS,GD P-40,I
14. K	60	f	DFS(75)	P2,E	---	P-20,E	OS no effect P2,P-20,E
15. G	60	m	DFS(74)	P2,I	---	P-40,I	ODS +
16. vS	52	m	P2	DFS(73)	P-20	---	ODS +
17. dS	64	f	GS,GD	DFS(73)	P-20,E	---	ODS +

12, 15 and 17 o'clock on the second and fourth day after cessation of therapy.

Phase 2: Two diurnal-curves with conventional therapy: pilocarpine 1, 2 cr 4% was given four times daily and in a few cases epinephrine and/or acetazolamide was added if needed to provide adequate control. Some patients were treated with a combination of glaucostat®/glaucadrine®. These IOP day-curves were made on the 7th and 9th day after the beginning of therapy.

Phase 3: Detailed verbal and printed instruction for the patients concerning the Ocusert handling.

Phase 4: IOP diurnal-curves with Ocusert beginning on the second day after cessation of therapy. In the patients of protocol 1 Ocusert was given to one eye, while the fellow eye remained on eye-drops (pilocarpine in most cases), again in addition with epinephrine and/or acetazolamide if needed. IOP diurnal-curves were made of both eyes to compare the Ocusert effect with conventional methods of therapy on the 1st, 3rd and 7th day of the 1st week and on the 6th and 7th day of the 2nd week. When reduction of IOP was satisfactory, patients were examined every 3 months. In the patients of protocol 2 we tried to evaluate the effect of pilocarpine and Ocusert on IOP after a filtrating operation. Some patients were treated with Ocusert in both eyes.

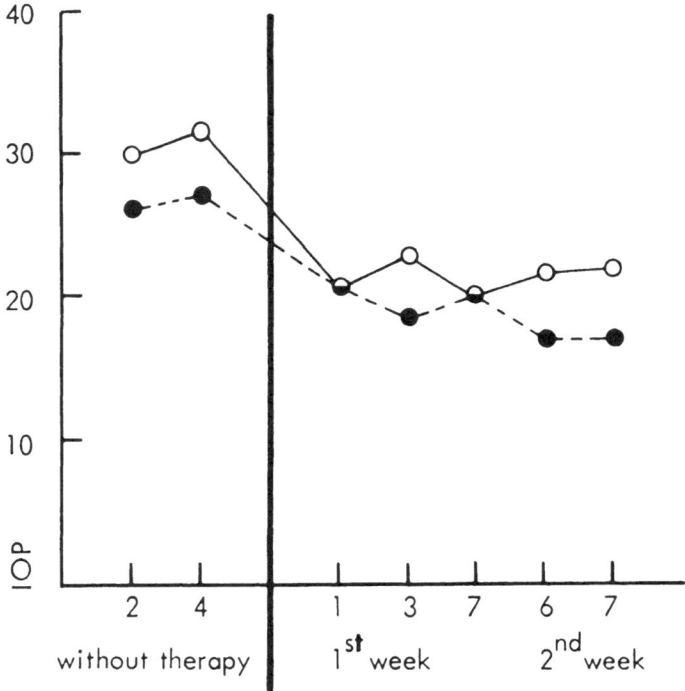

Fig. 2. Patient no. 2; average IOP 2 and 4 days after cessation of therapy. One eye treated with Ocusert P-40 (o), fellow eye with pilocarpine 2% eye-drops four times daily (•).

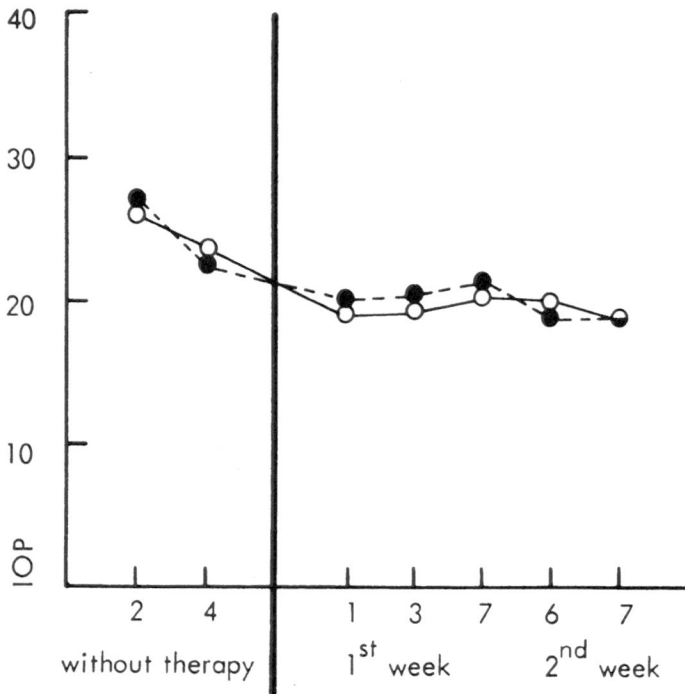

Fig. 3. Patient no. 3; average IOP 2 and 4 days after cessation of therapy. One eye treated with Ocusert P 20 (o), fellow eye with pilocarpine 2% eye-drops four times daily (●).

Originally 24 patients entered the study. Two of them were excluded because their IOP were consistently less than 22 mm Hg. appl. One patient left the study because of pain after inserting the Ocusert and preferred eye-drop medication. He noticed no congestion or blurring, so that it seems unlikely that there was leakage as reported by Lee et al. (1975). Of the remaining 21 patients 9 were female and the average age was 64 years.

The diagnoses were as follows: established glaucoma 15, of which 1 had pigmentary glaucoma; glaucoma suspect 4; low tension glaucoma 1, and secondary glaucoma 1.

The tables 1 to 6 describe the type of glaucoma of the 21 patients, their prestudy medication, the eye or eyes in which they had Ocusert and the effect of the therapy on IOP (control). No effect P2, P-20 means that neither pilocarpine 2% eye-drops, nor Ocusert P-20 had a significant effect on IOP.

Results

IOP:
— the 21 patients used Ocusert for a period varying from 4 to 24 weeks. Most of the patients used Ocusert for more than 12 weeks.

52

- 14 of the 21 patients have used Ocusert with a satisfactory reduction of IOP. This means that the IOP reduction was as substantial as that of pilocarpine eye-drops and that the IOP was brought down to an acceptable level (table 1, 2, 4, 5).
- in 5 of these 14 patients epinephrine eye-drops were added to Ocusert. The combination was well tolerated and the additive hypotensive effect comparable with that of pilocarpine and epinephrine eye-drops.

TABLE 6. Clinical data of 4 patients with primary established glaucoma, prestudy medication, current therapy and effect. For abbreviations used see table 1

PRIMARY (ESTABLISHED) GLAUCOMA	{ wide angle 3 { narrow angle – { chronic narrow angle 1

OCUSERT IN THE OPERATED EYE

PAT.	AGE	SEX	PRESTUDY MEDICATION		OCUSERT		CONTROL
			OD	OS	OD	OS	ODS
18. V	62	f	GS,GD	DFS(72) GS,GD	GS,GD	P-20,I	OS no effect P-20,I
19. L	62	f	DFS(73)	SCHEIE (71)	P2,E AC	P-20,E	no effect P-20, P2,E
20. E	74	f	DFS(73) P2	DFS(73)	P-20	– – –	no effect P-20, P2
21. K	24	m	DFS(73)	DFS(74) revocation	P-20,I AC	P-20,I	OD + OS no effect P-20,I

TABLE 7. Functional and proportional parameters of the Ocusert P-20 and P-40 system

FUNCTIONAL PARAMETERS:	P 20	P 40
Pilocarpine delivery rate	20 mcg/h	40 mcg/h
Therapeutic lifetime	7 days	7 days
Total 7 day delivery of pilocarpine	3,4 mg	6,7 mg
Pilocarpine content	5 mm	11 mg
PROPORTIONAL PARAMETERS:		
Length	13,4 mm	13,0 mm
Width	5,7 mm	5,5 mm
Thickness	0,3 mm	0,5 mm
Weight	19,0 mg	29,0 mg

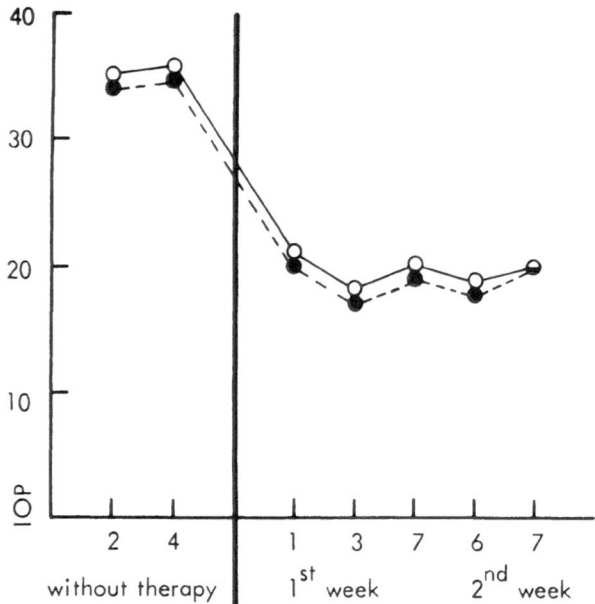

Fig. 4. Patient no. 4; average IOP 2 and 4 days after cessation of therapy. One eye treated with Ocusert P-20 (o), fellow eye with pilocarpine 2% eye-drops four times daily (•) and acetazolamide 125 mp, three times daily.

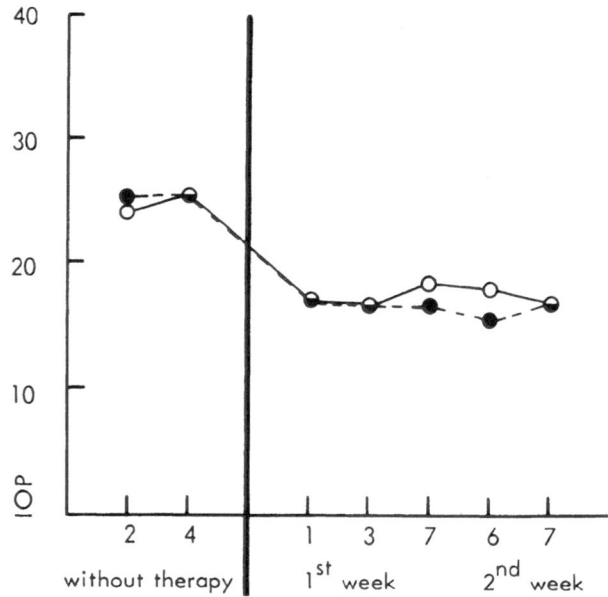

Fig. 5. Patient no. 5; average IOP 2 and 4 days after cessation of therapy. One eye treated with Ocusert P-20 (o), fellow eye with pilocarpine 1% eye-drops four times daily (•).

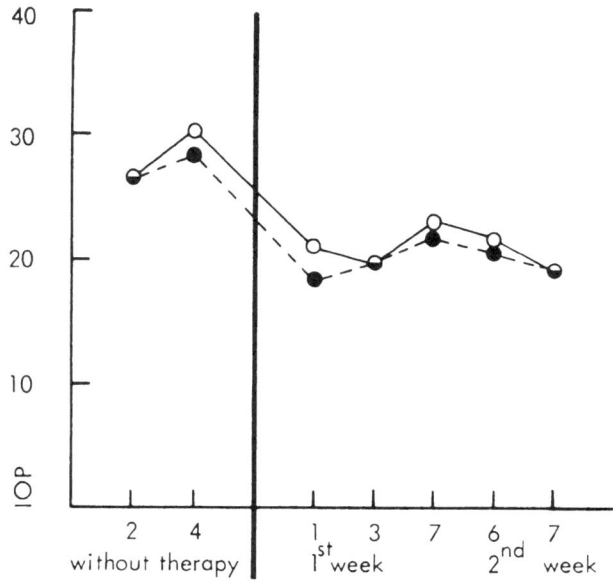

Fig. 6. Patient no. 6; average IOP 2 and 4 days after cessation of therapy. One eye treated with Ocusert P-40 (o), fellow eye with pilocarpine 2% eye-drops four times daily (•).

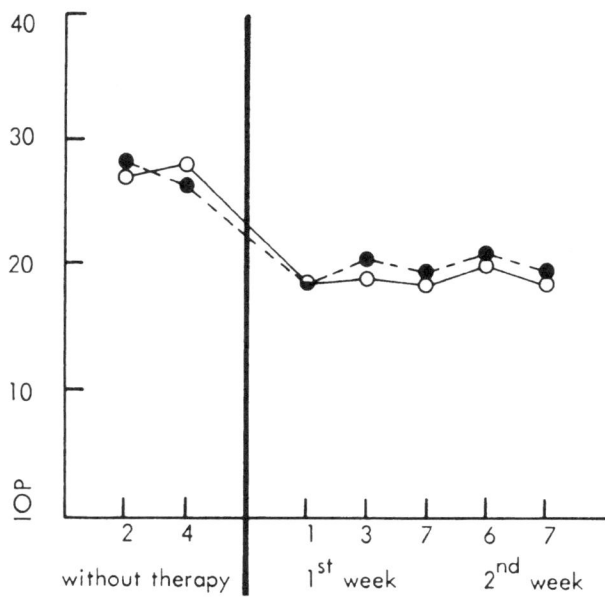

Fig. 7. Patient no. 7; average IOP 2 and 4 days after cessation of therapy. One eye treated with Ocusert P-20 (o), fellow eye treated with pilocarpine 2% eye-drops four times daily (•).

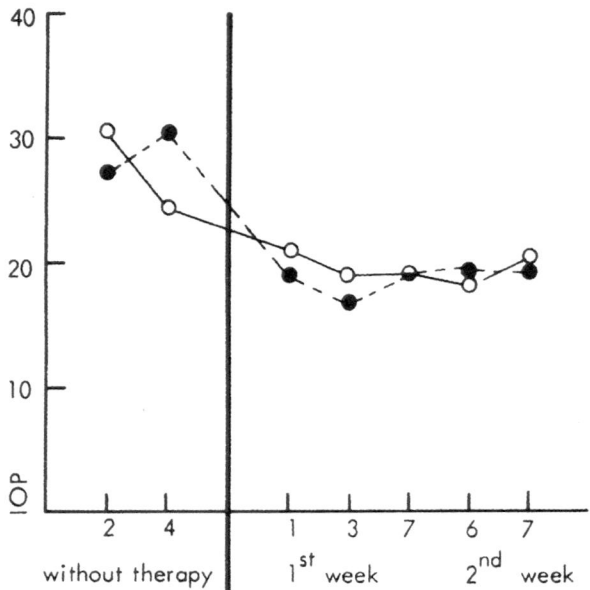

Fig. 8. Patient no. 10; average IOP 2 and 4 days cessation of therapy. One eye treated with Ocusert P-20 (o) and Isopto Epinal 1% fellow eye treated with glaucostat®/ glaucadrine® (●).

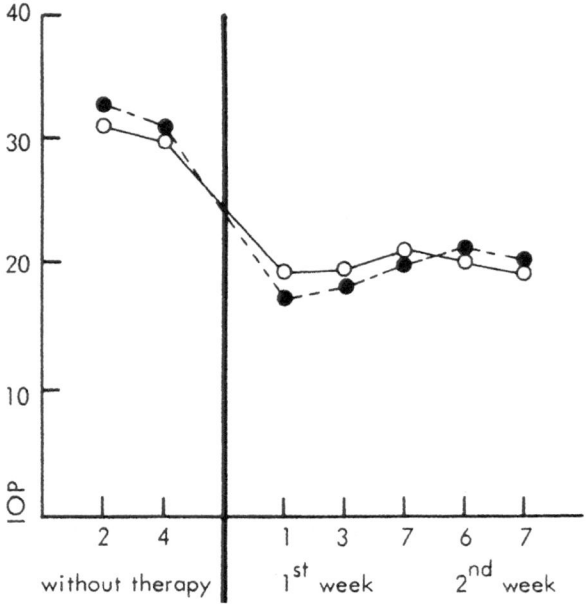

Fig. 9. Patient no. 12; average IOP 2 and 4 days after cessation of therapy. One eye treated with Ocusert P-40 and Isopto Epinal 1% (o), fellow eye treated with glaucostat®/glaucadrine® (●).

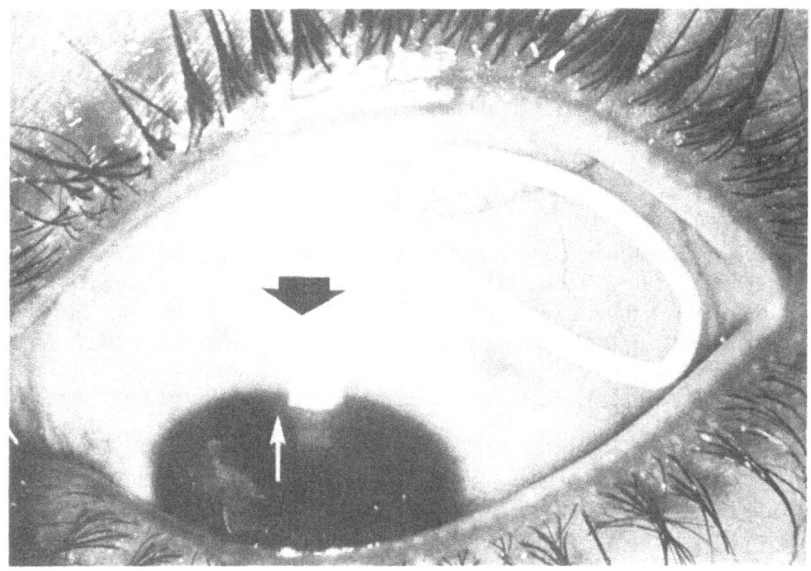

Fig. 10. Ocusert in an operated eye (double flap Scheie). Black arrow indicating filtrating bleb. White arrow indicating iridectomy.

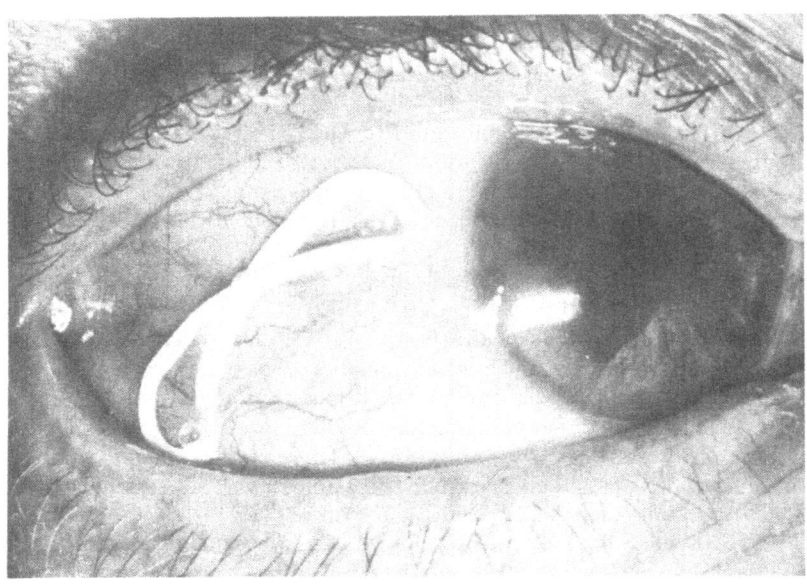

Fig. 11. '8'-formation of Ocusert.

57

- in 5 of 21 patients Ocusert pilocarpine did not produce any or only slight reduction of IOP. This concerns 4 patients where Ocusert was placed in the operated eye and 1 patient with low tension glaucoma. These 5 eyes did not react to conventional application of miotic eye-drops. They show that Ocusert cannot do anything more than eye-drops as far as the average reduction of IOP is concerned (table 3, 6). They also show that Ocusert is well tolerated in an operated eye (double flap Scheie). (Fig. 10).
- in 2 of 21 patients (one eye operated, Ocusert in the fellow eye) the IOP remained high with Ocusert and additional therapy, showing that Ocusert did no more than eye-drops (table 5).
- 10 of these 21 patients had Ocusert in one eye and pilocarpine or glaucostat® eye-drops in the fellow eye, or in combination with epinephrine; 9 of these with a satisfactory reduction of IOP (see Fig. 1 to 9).

Side effects

Of the 21 patients 2 never lost the Ocusert-module, 3 noticed frequent '8'-formation, 1 had a corneal erosion, 2 had a subconjunctival bleeding and in 1 patient the Ocusert-module frequently displaced to the pupil.

We noticed more '8'-formation and device loss, when the patient had rigid eyelids and/or a narrow interpalpebral fissure. We could not find a correlation between the tear production (Schirmer-test) and some ocular discomfort in the first weeks, when the patient had to get accustomed to the Ocusertmodule.

We observed no leakage, infection or an adverse effect of '8'-formation on IOP.

Conclusion

- It can be concluded that pilocarpine in Ocusert gives the same reduction of IOP as pilocarpine in eye-drops. With regard to the level of IOP reduction Ocusert does nothing more or less than eye-drops.
- If pilocarpine eye-drops have no effect it makes no sense to prescribe Ocusert.
- From this investigation no conclusion can be drawn about the reduction of IOP during the night.
- There were no serious side effects.
- The ocular tolerance and patient compliance were very good. With the exception of one, all patients preferred Ocusert to eye-drops. The main reason being that they did not have to administer their eye-drops four times daily.
- Induced myopia and miosis were not measured but it is well known from the literature that these are less than with pilocarpine eye-drops (Place, 1975; Leydecker, 1975). The complaints of the patients about twilight vision and blurring with Ocusert were much less than in the case after miotic eye-drops.
- The main advantage of Ocusert is the constant delivery rate of pilocar-

pine in which the side effects of the overdose-underdose regime are avoided.

- Loss of device and '8'-formation occurred quite often, usually in the same patients (Fig. 11). We observed no adverse effect on the IOP of '8'-formation. We noticed no leakage and only in one case the Ocusert was dislocated to the centre of the cornea hindering vision.
- A substantial disadvantage of Ocusert is the price. It will cost 10 to 15 times as much as conventional pilocarpine eye-drop therapy. There are, however, several indications where Ocusert is to be preferred to eye-drops, notwithstanding the price.

Summary

21 patients were treated with the Ocusert pilocarpine system for a period varying from 4 to 24 weeks. 10 of these patients had Ocusert in one eye and pilocarpine or glaucostat® eye-drops in the fellow eye, or in combination with epinephrine, 9 of them with a satisfactory reduction of IOP (see Fig. 1 to 9). With regard to the level of IOP reduction it can be said that pilocarpine in Ocusert gives the same reduction as pilocarpine eye-drops. From this investigation no conclusions can be drawn about the reduction of IOP during the night. We saw no serious side effects. The main advantage of the Ocusert system is the constant and continuous delivery of pilocarpine in which the side effects of the overdose-underdose regime are avoided.

REFERENCES

Armaly, M.F. & K.R. Rao. The effect of pilocarpine Ocusert on ocular pressure. In: Symposium Ocular Therapy, 6. Ed. I.H. Leopold, Mosby, St. Louis 80, (1973).

Armaly, M.F. & K.R. Rao. The effect of pilocarpine Ocusert with different release rates on ocular pressure. *Invest. Ophthal.* 12, 491, (1973).

Bucci, M.G. & E. Romani. L'Ocusert-pilocarpina nella terapia del glaucoma. *Boll. Oculist.* 51, 293, (1972).

Draeger, J., G. Haselmann & B. Weber. Der Einfluss von Pilocarpin auf die Kammerwasserdynamik bei Verwendung von Medikamententrägern mit Kontinuierlicher Abgaberate. *Klin. Mbl. Augenheilkunde* 167, 527, (1975).

Drance, S.M., D.W.A. Mitchell, M. Schulzer. The duration of action of pilocarpine Ocusert on intraocular pressure in man. *Canad. J. Ophthal.* 10, 450 (1975).

Friederich, R.I. The pilocarpine Ocusert: a new drug delivery system. *Ann. Ophthal.* 6, 1279, (1974).

Heilmann, K. & U. Sinz. Ocusert, ein neuartiges Medikamententrägersystem für die Glaukombehandlung. I. Mitteilung. *Klin. Mbl. Augenheilk.* 165, 519, (1974).

Heilmann, K. & U. Sinz. Idem II. Mitteilung. *Klin. Mbl. Augenheilk.* 166, 289, (1975).

Heilmann, K. & U. Sinz. Idem III. Mitteilung. *Klin. Mbl. Augenheilk.* 167, 534, (1975).

Krieglstein, G.K. Pilocarpin-Ocusert P-40 bei Glaukomproblemfällen. *Klin. Mbl. Augenheilk.* 167, 55, (1975).

Lee, P., Shen, Yeong-Tai & M. Eberle. The long-acting Ocusert-pilocarpine system in the management of glaucoma. *Invest. Ophthal.* 14, 43, (1975).

Leydhecker, W., S. Trapp, D. Linnert & M. Gail. Ocusert Pilocarpin bei Glaucoma simplex. *Klin. Mbl. Augenheilk.* 166, 285, (1975).

Lienert, F., H. Busse. Ein Jahr Erfahrungen mit Pilocarpin-Ocusert in der Glaukombehandlung. *Klin. Mbl. Augenheilk.* 167, 870, (1975).

Macoul, K.L. & D. Pavan-Langston. Pilocarpine Ocusert system for sustained controle of ocular hypertension. *Arch. Ophthal.* 93, 587, (1975).

Place, V.A., M. Fisher, S. Herbst, L. Gordon & R.C. Merrill. Comparative pharmacologic effects of pilocarpine administered to normal subjects by eyedrops or by ocular therapeutic systems. *Amer. J. Ophthal.* 80, 706, (1975).

Quigley, H.A., I.P. Pollack & T.S. Harbin Jr. Pilocarpine Ocuserts. Long-term clinical trials and selected pharmacodynamics. *Arch. Ophthal.* 93, 771, (1975).

Richardson, K.T. Ocular microtherapy. *Arch. Ophthal.* 93, 74, (1975).

Richardson, K.T. Dynamic principles of membranes and clinical pharmacology. In: Symposium on glaucoma. Trans. New Orleans Acad. Ophthal., Mosby, St. Louis. 31, (1975).

Richardson, K.T. Membrane-controlled drugdelivery. In: Symposium on glaucoma. Trans. New Orleans Acad. Ophthal., Mosby, St. Louis. 50, (1975).

Worthen, D.M., T.J. Zimmerman & C.A. Wind. An evaluation of the pilocarpine Ocusert. *Invest. Ophthal.* 13, 296, (1974).

Author's address:
Eye Clinic of the University of Amsterdam
Wilhelmina Gasthuis
Eerste Helmerstraat 104
Amsterdam
The Netherlands

LONG-TERM USE OF OCUSERT®

K. HEILMANN

(Munich)

I. GENERAL

Ocusert® (pilocarpine) Pilo-20 / Pilo-40 is one of several ocular Therapeutic Systems and has been tested clinically since 1972. As most clinical trials were undertaken for a relatively short period, my aim was to obtain information − which has hitherto been lacking − on the effects of continuous release of a substance to the eye over extended periods. It is understandable that such a clinical study can only be carried out with a small collective of patients because they have to be kept together for years under continuous observation. In the clinical assessment, the membrane unit was the unknown component to be tested and pilocarpine the known antiglaucomatous substance. Such an important problem as the question whether a consistent IOP is more suitable for maintaining morphological structures (papilla) and sensoric functions (visual field) was not the object of this investigation. The following aspect were especially taken into consideration:
− The effect on the IOP, on the pupil and on accommodation during the 7 days functional life of the Ocusert unit,
− the effects of continuous controlled drug delivery on long-term use,
− the patient acceptance and patient satisfaction compared to conventional dosage forms.

It is to be hoped that the use of the Ocusert unit and the dissemination of ocular Therapeutic Systems will be facilitated by some findings which are of practical importance and which have arisen from the use of Ocusert in the same patients for 30 months now.

II. EFFECT ON THE IOP, ON THE PUPIL AND ON ACCOMMODATION DURING THE 7 DAYS FUNCTIONAL LIFE OF THE OCUSERT UNIT

With both the Pilo-20 and the Pilo-40 units it is possible to reduce IOP in patients with open-angle glaucoma to a clinically relevant extent round-the-clock for at least 7 days. The effect on the IOP is comparable to the treatment with pilocarpine eye-drops (2%) four times a day. During conventional treatment a total of 28 mg pilocarpine is released in 7 days, with the Ocusert unit 3.4 mg (Pilo-20) or 6.7 mg (Pilo-40) is sufficient to produce the same pressure reducing effect. After insertion of the unit, the substance diffuses first with increased rate through the rate-controlling membrane until, after a few hours, the steady state situation is reached and pilocarpine is released in zero-order pattern. The initially higher drug delivery also results in a more intense effect on the pupil and on the ciliary muscle; if the weekly changing of the unit is done in the evening, then this process occurs in the early hours of the night and is thus unnoticed by the patient.

During treatment with Ocusert — apart from the beginning and end of the therapy — pupil size corresponds to a value which would be recorded 14 hours after the application of pilocarpine in oil, while the increase in myopia is comparable to a value registered 2 to 3 hours after the use of pilocarpine drops. These values were obtained in relatively old patients. In young people the differences may be more pronounced, the fact that miosis and accommodative myopia are extremely constant being a particular advantage.

III. EFFECTS OF CONTINUOUS CONTROLLED DRUG DELIVERY ON LONG-TERM USE

We do not know the effect of continuous release of an active substance on the structures of the inner-eye. One effect of zero-order release pattern for example may be the continuous contraction of the longitudinal fibres of the ciliary muscle, so that the question arises whether morphological changes occur in the course of time under the influence of a substance when constantly supplied. Such a conversion could possibly lead to the state where the miotic substance loses its effect with time, on the other hand a situation could be created in which all further use of a miotic to improve outflow facility would be superfluous. Such ideas are conceivable, their validity is provable only on the basis of long-term clinical observations exactly carried out on the same patient collective.

From the diurnal curves (Fig. 1) carried out over 24 months it can be seen that the IOP is lowered to a good to very good extent. From the regression curve (Fig. 2) it appears that in the course of 6 months considerable pressure changes may occur. It is not yet possible to establish how long and how high IOP may rise before an effect is to be considered lacking. This applies to patients 3 and 9 (left eyes). The omission test (Fig. 3) performed with placebo units show that the effect of IOP reduction remains reversible; except for patient 18, the rise in IOP recurred within 24 hours. At the present time, the conclusion can be drawn that the continuous application of pilocarpine has not led either to clinically recognisable changes in morphological structures or to a noticeable decreasing sensitivity to the drug so far.

IV. THE PATIENT ACCEPTANCE AND PATIENT SATISFACTION COMPARED TO CONVENTIONAL DOSAGE FORMS

Since previous medical therapy for the eye consisted of the application of drops, oil or ointment, the insertion of a membrane unit, i.e. a solid body, is a change for the patient as well as for the ophthalmologist. The results so far

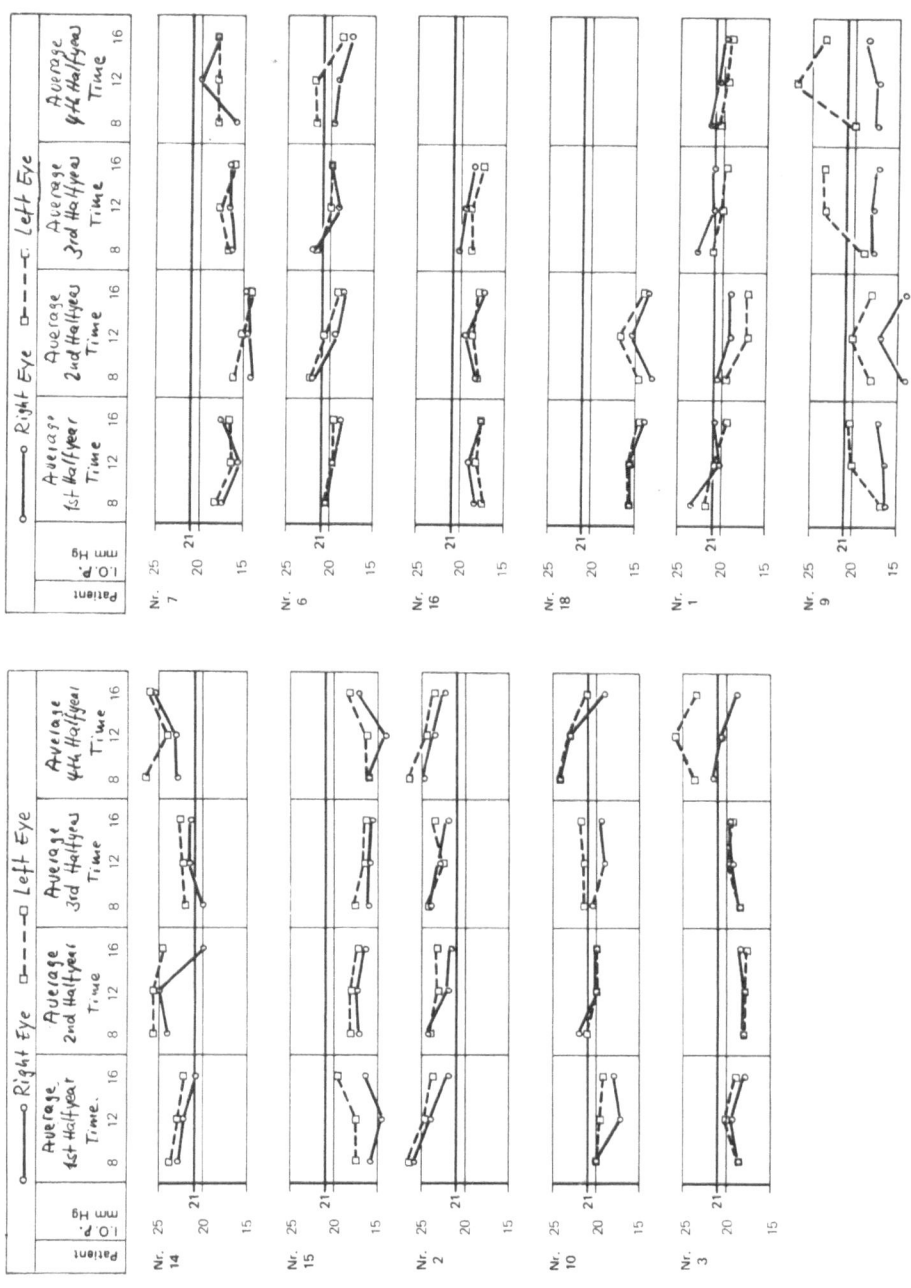

Fig. 1. Intraocular Pressure. Diurnal curves.

63

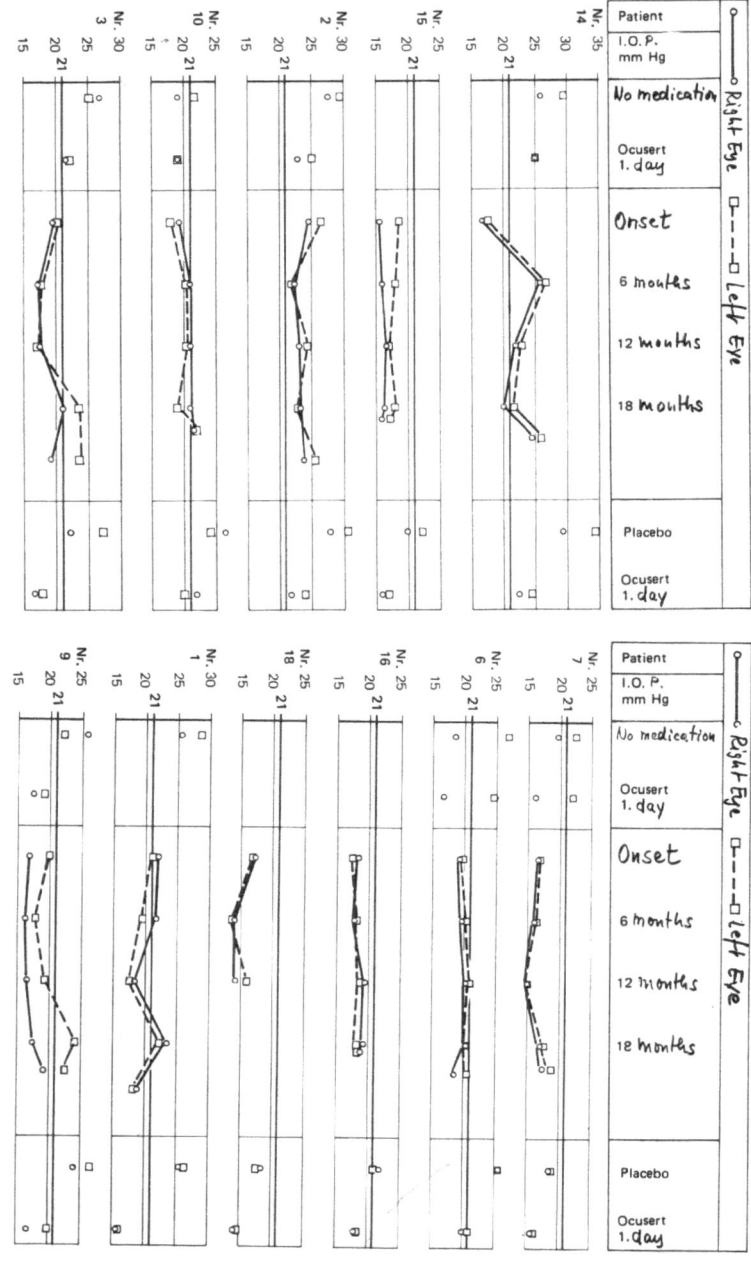

Fig. 2. Intraocular Pressure. Regression curve over the total duration of investigation (Average values of the day).

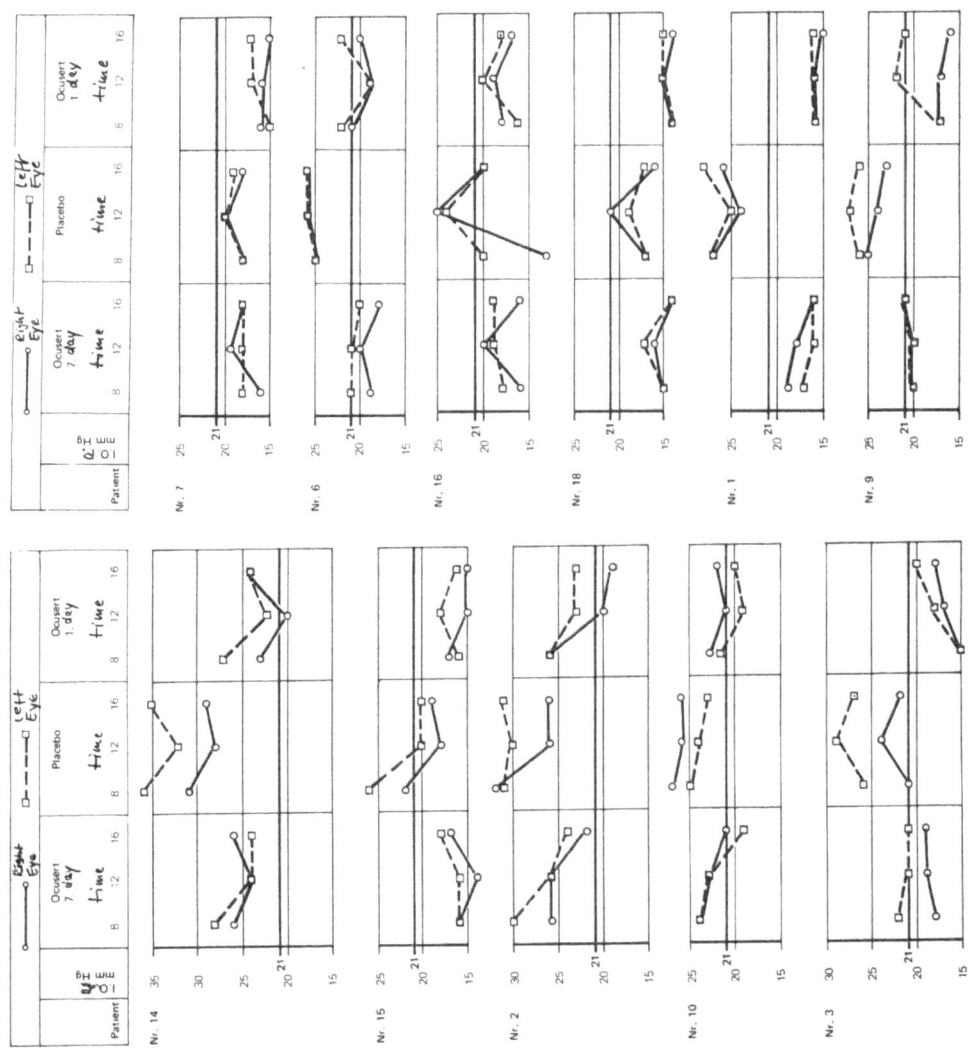

Fig. 3. Omission test. Intraocular Pressure. Diurnal Curves.

65

show that the success or failure of the patient in the use of Ocusert is closely related to the personal attitude of the doctor to this novel form of drug application. If the doctor has already decided after one day that this kind of treatment is unsuitable for a patient because of frequent membrane loss, this attempt must be considered useless. In our experience, the patient should wear Ocusert for at least two or three weeks, intensive care of the patient during that time being essential. Within a few weeks, the eye seems to become adapted to the 'foreign body' and patients report that the difficulties cease completely with increasing practice. If then at a later date the unit is occasionally reported to be lost, or distortion or leakage develops, this event seems to be related to a certain membrane itself.

The patients we have treated with Ocusert unanimously state that 'not having to have drops any more' means for them especially not being constantly reminded of the disease. Anyone who has glaucoma patients constantly under his care can assess the significance of this statement. Since chronic open-angle glaucoma is a symptomless disease that in no way impairs the patient's rhythm of life at first, it is usually difficult to make him realise the necessity for a treatment with which considerable discomforts are associated. Furthermore it is a natural duty for the physician not only to treat the disease, but also to make the treatment easier and bearable for the patient.

While the measurable effects of Ocusert in the literature are in good agreement with each other regarding IOP, pupil size and myopia, the results in relation to the practical use of the system vary. For the interpretation of the various communications it is necessary to know whether or not the doctor himself has any experience with the unit and knowledge of the principles of constant drug release and whether he has initiated the patient into the management of the unit for a certain time. Concerning patient acceptance and experience, such important information as whether these data are obtained from patients with experience in conventional treatment with eye-drops or whether the use of Ocusert was the first treatment attempted at all is usually lacking in the literature. A patient with years of experience with eye-drops will assess such factors as foreign body-feeling, miosis and accommodative myopia completely differently from a patient who is not familiar with such effects.

V. CONCLUSIONS

From the results in the literature and our own experience over 2½ years it is established that there is no particular indication for ocular Therapeutic Systems, and that the constant and, in comparison to the effects of conventional dosage forms very slight effects on the pupil and accommodation as well as the novel effect of dissociating the patient from his disease are the prominent features of membrane controlled drug delivery. Ocusert is suitable for the treatment of all glaucoma patients. At the present time it is only available with pilocarpine as active substance, which means some limitation. Ocusert with pilocarpine is not suitable for all types of glaucoma, because the use of miotics e.g. in inflammatory secondary glaucoma is contra-indicated. Ocusert with pilocarpine can also be used in patients with chronic angle-closure glaucoma if particular circumstances make surgical intervention impossible. According to more recent investigations the use of pilocarpine in angle-closure glaucoma flattens the anterior chamber and narrows the chamber angle, an effect which is less pronounced with pilocarpine released constantly in small rates. The patient should, however, be particularly familiar with the handling of the unit and convince himself of its presence in the conjunctival cul-de-sac at regular intervals. The doctor also has a particular responsibility in such a case.

Even after many years of clinical experience with the Therapeutic System Ocusert it is at this time not possible fully to recognise potential undesirable side effects. This applies in the same way to the positive effects of the treatment which increase with increasing experience. Altogether the clinical results are extremely encouraging: Ocusert is a new approach to treating glaucoma, after years of stagnation, medical therapy has really received a new impetus.

REFERENCES

Armaly, M.F. & K.R. Rao: The effect of pilocarpine Ocusert with different release rates on ocular pressure. *Invest. Ophthal.* 12, *491* (1973).

Armaly, M.F. & K.R. Rao: The effect of pilocarpine Ocusert on ocular pressure. In: 'Symposium on Ocular Therapy' Vol. 6 (I.H. Leopold, ed.) Mosby, St. Louis 1973.

Bucci, M.G. & E. Romani: Ocusert-Pilocarpine in glaucoma therapy. (Italian, English translation.) *Boll. Oculist.* 51, *293* (1972).

Frauenfelder, F.T. & C. Hanna: Ophthalmic drug delivery systems. *Surv. Ophthal.* 18, *292* (1974).

Frauenfelder, F.T.: A new drug delivery system. Ophthal. Digest, Nov. 1974, 27.

Friederich, R.I.: The pilocarpine Ocusert: a new drug delivery system. *Ann. Ophthal.* 6, *1279* (1974).

Heilmann, K.: Medikamentöse Glaukomtherapie. Enke, Stuttgart 1974.

Heilmann, K. & U. Sinz: Ocusert, ein neuartiges Medikamententrägersystem für die Glaukombehandlung, 1. *Mitteilung. Klin. Mbl. Augenheilk.* 165, *519* (1974).

Heilmann, K. & U. Sinz: Ocusert, ein neuartiges Medikamententrägersystem für die Glaukombehandlung. 2. *Mitteilung. Klin. Mbl. Augenheilk.* 166, *289* (1975).

Heilmann, K.: Ocusert, ein neuartiges Medikamententrägersystem für die Glaukombehandlung. 3. *Mitteilung. Klin. Mbl. Augenheilk.* 167, *534* (1975).

Heilmann, K.: Ocusert, ein neuartiges Medikamententrägersystem für die Glaukombehandlung. 4. Mitteilung. (in press).

Heilmann, K.: Therapeutische Systeme. Konzept und Realisation organspezifischer Arzneiverabreichung. Enke, Stuttgart 1977.

Holland, M.G.: Autonomic drugs in ophthalmology: some problems and promises. Section 1: Directly and indirectly acting parasympathomimetic drugs. Ann. Ophthal. 6, *447* (1974).

Krieglstein, G.K.: Pilocarpin-Ocusert P-40 bei Glaukomproblemfällen. *Klin. Mbl. Augenheilk.* 167, *55* (1975).

Lerman, S: Simulated sustained release pilocarpine therapy. *Ann. Ophthal.* 2, *437* (1970).

Lerman, S. & B. Reininger: Simulated sustained release pilocarpine therapy and aqueous humor dynamics. *Canad. J. Ophthal.* 6, *14* (1971).

Lerman, S.: Prolonged release medication in the treatment of eye disease. *Israel J. med. Sci.* 8, *1402* (1972).

Leydhecker, W. & S. Trapp, D. Linnert, M. Gail: Ocusert Pilocarpin bei Glaucoma Simplex. *Klin. Mbl. Augenheilk.* 166, *285* (1975).

Place, V.A. & J.W. Shell: Ocusert Pilo 20 Pilo 40 (pilocarpine) ocular therapeutic systems: Clinical Experiences. Scientific Exhibit New Orleans Academy of Ophthalmology, 23rd Ann. Symp. New Orleans (La.) 1974.

67

Richardson, K.T.: Pharmacology and Toxicology. *Arch. Ophthal. (Chic.)* 89, *65* (1973).

Sauer, D.W.: Effects of different temporal patterns of pilocarpine release on intra-ocular pressure in patients with ocular hypertension. Association for Research in Vision and Ophthalmology, Ann. Meet., Sarasota, May 1973.

Shell, J.W. & R.W. Baker: Temporal patterns of drug release from diffusional ocular delivery systems. Association for Research in Vision and Ophthalmology, Ann. Meet. Sarasota, May 1973.

Shell, J.W.: A new method of administering ophthalmic drugs, Amer. Drug. 15. Sept. 1974, 44-45.

Shell, J.W. & R.W. Baker: Diffusional systems for controlled release of drugs to the eye. *Ann. Ophthalm.* 6, *1037* (1970).

Shell, J.W.: Ocular therapy by controlled drug delivery: *The Ocusert system. Ophthal. Surg.* 5, *73* (1974).

Worthen, D.M. & T.J. Zimmerman, C.A. Wind: An evaluation of the pilocarpine Ocusert. *Invest. Ophthal.* 13, *296* (1974).

Zimmerman, T.J. & D.M. Worthen: Clinical evaluation of an Ocusert-Pilocarpine delivery system. Association for Research in Vision and Ophthalmology, Ann. Meet. Sarasota, May 1973.

Author's address:
Hochkalterstrasse 8
D–8000 München
West Germany

ADRENERGIC INFLUENCES ON AQUEOUS HUMOUR DYNAMICS

G. PATERSON

(London)

With the stimulus that has evolved from the considerable expansion in research in brain monoamines and the continuing growth in knowledge of peripheral autonomic innervation, it has become clear that even the relatively uncomplicated concept of peripheral adrenergic neuro-effector cell junctional transmission must constantly be revised.

THE ADRENERGIC INNERVATION OF INTRA-OCULAR STRUCTURES

Although a considerable amount of effort has gone into the mapping out of adrenergic nerve pathways to structures contiguous with the anterior chamber the physiological significance of this innervation has, in all but a few instances, eluded satisfactory explanation. One of the more successful techniques for demonstrating the presence of adrenergic nerves has been the fluorescent histochemical method of Falck and Hillarp (Falck, 1962; Falck, Hillarp, Thieme & Torp, 1962). Basically the method consists of sectioning a tissue under cryotome conditions. The sections are then freeze-dried and heated in formaldehyde vapour at 80° C for one hour. It is then possible to visualise in an ultraviolet microscope a yellow-green fluorescence which corresponds to the localisation of adrenergic nerves. The method has been used with success by Ehinger (1966) with sections of eyes of primates. Adrenergic nerves have been identified in the ciliary processes, in the iris and in the ciliary trabeculae, although not in the scleral trabeculae. Some sparse innervation of the ciliary muscle could also be demonstrated. In electron microscope studies Uusitalo & Palkama (1971) were able to establish that in the ciliary processes there was direct contact between adrenergic nerves and the secretory cells of the ciliary epithelia of rabbits' eyes.

ADRENOTROPIC RECEPTORS

It has been firmly established that noradrenaline is the main peripheral adrenergic neural transmitter in mammals (von Euler, 1946 et seq.) and that transmission is mediated by adrenotropic receptors (see: Ahlquist, 1966; Paterson, 1966; Blaschko & Muscholl, 1972; Burnstock & Costa, 1975). These receptors have been subclassified on the basis of agonist and antagonist selectivity. In effect three forms of receptors have been identified and have been designated α-, β_1- and β_2-adrenoceptors. The α-receptors can be distinguished from the β-receptors on the basis that noradrenaline and adrenaline are much more effective than isoprenaline at α-receptor sites. Also, specific antagonists such as phentolamine and phenoxybenzamine will block agonist activity at α-receptor sites, but have no β-receptor blocking activity. Similarly, β-receptors can be identified by the much greater activity of isoprenaline at these receptors than is found with adrenaline or noradrenaline. Again, β-receptor blocking drugs such as propranolol and oxprenolol have specific actions at these sites. The subdivision of β-receptors into β_1- and β_2-receptors is a more recent and controversial concept. This differentiation is also relative and not as absolute as that between α- and β-receptors. Agonists have been synthesized which are relatively specific for β_2-receptors and antagonists which are relatively specific for either β_1- or β_2-receptors.

Levy (1976) has made an exhaustive analysis of the reactions of receptors present in a number of tissues and was able to confirm, on the basis of the agonist activity of salbutamol, adrenaline and noradrenaline, that, in vitro at least, a clear difference existed between β_1- and β_2-receptors. The β_1-receptors which were characterised in the heart and fat depots were more responsive to noradrenaline than to adrenaline and at these sites the antagonistic action of practolol against isoprenaline was high (pA_2 of 6.6 to 6.8). On the other hand, the β_2-receptors found in the smooth muscle of the bronchial tree and in vascular smooth muscle were more sensitive to adrenaline than to noradrenaline and the antagonistic action of practolol against isoprenaline was relatively low (pA_2 of 4.7 to 5.1). Salbutamol (Brittain, Farmer, Jack, Martin & Simpson, 1968; Cullum, Farmer, Jack & Levy, 1969) was also confirmed to be more effective on those tissues containing β_2-receptors than on those containing β_1-receptors.

In ocular structures α-adrenoceptors have been shown to be present in the dilator pupillae muscle, in the blood vessels of the conjunctiva and sclera and in the levator palpebrae muscles. They have also been associated with the increased outflow facility from the anterior chamber seen with adrenaline and noradrenaline, the effects of which are blocked by the α-receptor blocking agent, phenoxybenzamine. β-adrenoceptor activity is involved in the relaxant effect of sympathomimetics on the sphincter pupillae of many species, a vasodilator action on most blood vessels, including those of the conjunctiva and a lowering of intra-ocular pressure caused mainly by a reduction in the formation of aqueous humour.

The effects on intra-ocular pressure of sympathomimetic drugs will thus be dictated by their selectivity at the different receptor sites and by the identity of the receptor population controlling the mechanism of action. If we take for instance isoprenaline, this drug will have as its main action an action on aqueous formation; however we cannot rule out α-receptor activity, as has been shown by Langham (1974) to be present when high concentrations are used. However, if the drug investigated is salbutamol, known for its very high selectivity for β-receptors, any effect mediated by α-receptors will be absent from its pattern of activity. It can then be reasonably assumed that effects seen involve β-receptor activation, an assumption which can be further tested by using a β-receptor blocking drug to abolish the action. This drug has been investigated in man, monkeys and rabbits (Paterson & Paterson, 1971, 1972) (Langham & Diggs, 1974) and causes a fall in intra-ocular pressure without affecting the α-receptor mediated dilatation of the pupil. Also propranolol blocks completely the effects of the salbutamol (Langham, 1974). Neither isoprenaline nor salbutamol has been proved to be useful in the long-term treatment of chronic simple glaucoma, isoprenaline because of its associated pronounced tachycardia seen even on topical application to the eye, (Ross & Drance, 1970), salbutamol because of the tachyphylaxis and hyperaemia which developed after some weeks of treatment (Paterson & Paterson, 1971). This tachyphylaxis to both α-receptor and β-receptor activation has been encountered frequently (Kitazawa, 1974) (Paterson & Conolly, 1970), (Langham, 1975), but appears to be more of a problem with drugs occupying β-receptors. No adequate explanation has yet been advanced for its occurrence.

UPTAKE OF SYMPATHOMIMETIC AMINES BY ADRENERGIC NERVES AND ASSOCIATED STRUCTURES

When an adrenergic nerve releases its transmitter, noradrenaline, this then crosses a junctional gap to occupy receptors situated either on or within the post-synaptic membrane. The junctional gap varies from tissue to tissue, being about 10 to 30 nm in the iris (Evans & Evans, 1964; Richardson, 1964; Uehara & Burnstock, 1972) and up to 400 nm in arteries (see Burnstock & Costa, 1975). After inducing its effect much of the noradrenaline (estimates vary between about 40 to 80 per cent., depending upon the tissue being examined) is recaptured by an active process present in the adrenergic nerve membrane (designated $Uptake_1$; Iversen, 1967, 1971). This uptake process will also reduce the effective concentration of many sympathomimetic drugs which diffuse into the junctional region either from the bloodstream or by other routes. $Uptake_1$ also exhibits a certain specificity; it will take up noradrenaline, adrenaline and dopamine, but will not transport isoprenaline or salbutamol. It is inhibited readily by a number of diverse substances, including cocaine, desipramine, nortriptyline, guanethidine and phenoxybenzamine. When $Uptake_1$ is inhibited by any of these substances the effects of adrenergic nerve stimulation or of applied noradrenaline or adrenaline are enhanced and prolonged. Such an increase in sensitivity is even more pronounced when adrenergic nerves are destroyed either as a result of chronic denervation or after chemical denervation by 6-hydroxydopamine. The potentiation of the action of topically applied adrenaline by guanethidine, (Paterson & Paterson, 1971), of noradrenaline and adrenaline by protriptyline, (Kitazawa & Langham, 1968; Langham & Carmel, 1968; Pollack, 1973) and the greatly increased effect of noradrenaline and adrenaline after sympathectomy with 6-hydroxydopamine (Holland & Wei, 1973; Kitazawa, Nose & Horie, 1973, 1975; Kitazawa, 1974) all depend on the inactivation of the $Uptake_1$ process.

A second inactivation process is also important in the removal of catecholamines from their sites of action. Some non-neural tissues, notably smooth muscle, will take up some sympathomimetics actively. This process is known as $Uptake_2$ and is responsible for the removal of about 20 per cent. of released noradrenaline at a smooth muscle neuro-effector junction.

It is not as specific as Uptake$_1$, isoprenaline being very effectively removed by its action. Again there are substances which will inhibit this extraneuronal uptake, among them β-oestradiol, normetanephrine and phenoxybenzamine.

It is likely that both Uptake$_1$ and Uptake$_2$ contribute to the low effectiveness of topically applied catecholamines. Certainly the inhibition or destruction of Uptake$_1$ leads to an enhancement of the actions of some of these amines. It is possible that inhibition of Uptake$_2$ might increase their effectiveness still further.

β-ADRENOCEPTOR BLOCKING DRUGS

A recent approach to the therapy of glaucoma has been the introduction of the β-adrenoceptor blocking drugs. (Phillips, Howitt & Rowlands, 1967; Vale, Gibbs & Phillips, 1972; Vale & Phillips, 1973; Bucci, Giraldi, Missiroli & Virno, 1968; Cote & Drance, 1968; Bonomi, Steindler & Chiricco, 1972). This series of drugs was only discovered some ten years after Ahlquist had advanced his theory of α- and β-receptors and did much to confirm this concept (Ahlquist, 1948; Powell & Slater, 1958). At the present time about eighty such compounds are known, of which fifteen are available clinically, with a further five undergoing clinical trials for the treatment of essential hypertension, angina pectoris and chronic simple glaucoma (Clark, 1976). The greater number of these do not distinguish between β_1- and β_2-receptors (e.g. propranolol, oxprenolol, sotalol, pindolol), but there are some which block β_1-receptors more readily than β_2-receptors (practolol, atenolol, metoprolol).

So far there appears to be no distinction between the two groups in respect of their abilities to lower intra-ocular pressure in normal subjects and glaucoma patients, which might indicate that the receptor which is relevant to the action is a β_1-receptor, but this would have to be researched further. As to where the receptor is situated can only be a matter of conjecture. The enigma has many similarities to that of the situation in the treatment of arterial hypertension with the β-adrenoceptor blocking agents.

REFERENCES

Ahlquist, R.P. A study of the adrenotropic receptors. *Amer. J. Physiol.*, 153, *586* (1948).

Ahlquist, R.P. The adrenergic receptor. *J. Pharm. Sci.* 55, *359* (1966).

Blaschko, H. & Muscholl, E., 'Catecholamines'. Springer-Verlag, Berlin (1972).

Bonomi, L., Steindler, P. & Chiriaco, G. Ocular effects of a new beta sympathicolytic drug, pindolol, (LB 46). *Ann. Ottalmol.* 98, *149* (1972).

Brittain, R.T., Farmer, J.B., Jack, D., Martin, L.E. & Simpson, W.T. α-[(*t*-Butylamino) methyl]-4-hydroxy-m-xylene-α^1; α^3-diol (AH 3365): a selective β-adrenergic stimulant. *Nature, (Lond.)*, 219, *862* (1968).

Bucci, M.G., Giraldi, J.P., Missiroli, A. & Virno, M. Local administration of propranolol in the glaucoma therapy. *Boll. Ocul.* 47, *51* (1968).

Burnstock, G. & Costa, M. 'Adrenergic Neurons'. Chapman and Hall, London (1975).

Clark, B.J. Pharmacology of beta-adrenoceptor blocking agents. In: 'Beta-adrenoceptor blocking agents: the pharmacological basis of clinical use'. (P.R. Saxena & R.P. Forsyth, editors). North Holland Publishing Co., Amsterdam (1976).

Cote, C. & Drance, S.M. The effect of propranolol on human intra-ocular pressure. *Can. J. Ophthalmol.* 3, *207* (1968).

Cullum, V.A., Farmer, J.B., Jack, D. & Levy, G.P. Salbutamol, a new, selective α-adrenoceptive receptor stimulant. *Br. J. Pharmac.*, 35, *141* (1969).

Ehinger, B. Ocular and orbital vegetative nerves. *Acta physiol. Scand.* 67, Supp. 268 (1966).

Evans, D.H.L. & Evans, E.M. The membrane relationships of smooth muscle: an electronmicroscope study. *J. Anat.*, 98, *37* (1964).

Euler, U.S. von. A specific sympathomimetic ergone in adrenergic nerve fibres (Sympathin) and its relation to adrenaline and noradrenaline. *Acta. physiol. Scand.*, 12, *73* (1946).

Falck, B. Observations on the possibilities of the cellular localisation of monoamines by a fluorescence method. *Acta physiol. Scand.*, 56, Supp. 197 (1962).

Falck, B., Hillarp, N-A., Thieme, G. & Torp, A. Fluorescence of catecholamines and related compounds condensed with formaldehyde. *J. Histochem. Cytochem.*, 10, *348* (1962).

Holland, M.G. & Mims, J.L. Anterior segment chemical sympathectomy by 6-hydroxydopamine. I. Effect on intra-ocular pressure and facility of outflow. *Invest. Ophthalmol.*, 10, *120* (1971).

Holland, M.G. & Wei, C. Chemical sympathectomy in glaucoma therapy: an investigation of alpha and beta adrenergic supersensitivity. *Ann. Ophthalmol.*, 5, *738* (1973).

Iversen, L.L. 'The uptake and storage of noradrenaline in sympathetic nerves'. University Press, Cambridge (1967).

Iversen, L.L. Role of transmitter uptake mechanisms in synaptic neurotransmission. *Br. J. Pharmac.*, 41, *571* (1971).

Kitazawa, Y. Discussion. In 'International Glaucoma Symposium, Albi' Marseilles. (R. Etienne & G.D. Paterson, editors) (1974).

Kitazawa, Y., Nose, H. & Horie, T. The effects of chemical sympathectomy on intra-ocular pressure in normal human subjects. *Acta Soc. Ophthalmol. Jap.*, 77, *1901* (1973).

Kitazawa, Y., Nose, H. & Horie, T. Chemical sympathectomy with 6-hydroxydopamine in the treatment of primary open-angle glaucoma. *Amer. J. Ophthalmol.* 79, *98* (1975).

Langham, M.E. The pharmacology of the adrenergic therapy of glaucoma. In: 'International Glaucoma Symposium, Albi'. (R. Etienne & G.D. Paterson, editors). Marseilles (1974).

Langham, M.E. Adrenergic tachyphylaxis in animal and human eyes. *Exp. Eye Res.*, 20, *174* (1975).

Langham, M.E. & Carmel, D.D. The action of protriptyline on adrenergic mechanisms in rabbit, primate and human eyes. *J. Pharmac. exp. Ther.*, 163, *368* (1968).

Langham, M.E. & Diggs, E. Beta-adrenergic responses in the eyes of rabbits, primates and man. *Exp. Eye Res.*, 19, *281* (1974).

Levy, G.P. Evidence obtained with selective agonists and antagonists in favour of the β_1- and β_2-adrenoceptor classification. Br. Pharm. Soc. Meeting, Oxford (1976).

Paterson, G. Sympathetic innervation and the actions of sympathomimetics. In: 'Drug Mechanisms in Glaucoma', (G. Paterson, S.J.H. Miller & G.D. Paterson, editors). Churchill, London (1966).

Paterson, G.D. & Paterson, G. A comparison of the ocular hypotensive actions of salbutamol and adrenaline in chronic simple glaucoma. *Postgrad. med. J.*, 47, March Supp. (Salbutamol), 122 (1971).

Paterson, G.D. & Paterson, G. Drug therapy of glaucoma. *Br. J. Ophthalmol.* 56, *288* (1972).

Paterson, J.W. & Conolly, M.E. The clinical pharmacology of inhaled isoprenaline. Proc. 12th Meeting Europ. Soc. Study Drug Toxicity. Excerpta Medica, Amsterdam (1970).

Phillips, C.I., Howitt, G. & Rowlands, D.J. Propranolol as ocular hypotensive agent. *Br. J. Ophthalmol.*, 51, *222* (1967).

Pollack, I.P. The effect of L-norepinephrine and adrenergic potentiators on the aqueous humour dynamics of man. *Am. J. Ophthalmol.*, 76, *641* (1973).

Powell, C.E. & Slater, I.H. Blocking of inhibitory adrenergic receptors by a dichloro-analogue of isoproterenol. *J. Pharmac. exp. Ther.*, 122, *480* (1958).

Richardson, K.C. The fine structure of the albino rabbit iris with special reference to the identification of adrenergic and cholinergic nerves and nerve endings in its intrinsic muscles. *Amer. J. Anat.*, 114, *173* (1964).

Ross, R.A. & Drance, S.M. Effects of topically applied isoproterenol on aqueous dynamics in man. *Arch. Ophthalmol.*, 83, *39* (1970).

Uehara, Y. & Burnstock, G. Postsynaptic specialisation of smooth muscle at close neuromuscular junctions in the guinea-pig sphincter pupillae. *J. Cell. Biol.*, 53, *849* (1972).

Uusitalo, R. & Palkama, A. Evidence for the nervous control of secretion in the ciliary processes. *Prog. Brain Res.*, 34, *513* (1971).

Vale, J., Gibbs, A.C.C. & Phillips, C.I. Topical propranolol and ocular tension in the human. *Br. J. Ophthalmol.*, 56, *770* (1972).

Vale, J. & Phillips, C.I. Practolol (Eraldin) eye drops as an ocular hypotensive agent. *Br. J. Ophthalmol.*, 57, *210* (1973).

Author's address:
c/o Moorfield Hospital
High Holborn
London WC1 V7AN
England

ADRENERGIC AND RELATED DRUGS

G.D. PATERSON

(London)

Interest in an effective non miotic therapy of open angle glaucoma has been renewed in recent years, largely as a result of the interesting new adrenergic drugs which have become available. These drugs have made it possible to reduce IOP quite profoundly, without the side effects of miosis, which are often disabling to the patient.

Adrenaline was the first adrenergic drug to be applied to the eye, and as far back as 1894 (Darier) it was found to lower the IOP. It was used in the treatment of glaucoma at the beginning of this century (Köllner), but its use was largely discontinued because of the inadvertent precipitation of acute attacks of angle closure. With the introduction of the gonioscope in 1940, and the subsequent classification of the glaucomas, interest was renewed in this drug, for treatment of the open angle forms of this disease. However adrenaline alone seldom reduces the IOP to a controlled limit of 20 mm.Hg. or less. Becker et al. (1961) demonstrated an average fall of 4.5 mm.Hg. after six months and on long term therapy one cannot expect a fall of more than 6mm.Hg. with this drug, using either the 1% or 2% solution. The hypotensive action of adrenaline lasts up to thirty hours with a maximum effect after six hours. Twice daily instillation is advised at twelve hourly intervals. The side effects include conjunctival hyperaemia, brow ache and the deposition of melanin in the conjunctiva. In aphakic subjects a non specific cystic maculopathy (Kolker 1968) can occur, but this is reversible and visual acuity returns to its former level when the adrenaline is discontinued.

The advantages of non miotic therapy stimulated research into the adrenergic field of drugs which has been directed along two main themes. Namely the search for either α or β agonists with a greater hypotensive effect than adrenaline, and secondly the combination of the use of adrenaline with a drug which will potentiate its action.

I. Other α and β agonists
    (a) Nor adrenaline
    (b) Isoprenaline
    (c) Salbutamol

II. Potentiators
    (a) Guanethidine
    (b) 6-Hydroxy dopamine
    (c) Protryptiline

NOR ADRENALINE

This drug has been investigated by Pollack & Rossi (1975). Using the free base in a 4% solution they demonstrated an average fall in IOP of 6mm.Hg, in eight eyes of patients with ocular hypertension, maintained over the 20 week period of study. An increase in the facility of outflow of aqueous humour was demonstrated in all the cases. Side effects were similar, brow ache and conjunctival hyperaemia, but less severe than those with adrenaline. Nor adrenaline 4% appears then to have an antihypertensive effect that is comparable to 1% adrenaline and because it seems to be more acceptable to the patient, should be regarded as a potentially useful drug.

ISOPRENALINE

Both Weekers, Collignon-Brach & Grieten (1966) and Ross & Drance (1970) have demonstrated the ocular hypotensive action of this drug. This was demonstrated in solutions of 5%, 2.5% and 1.25%. An early rise in IOP occurs followed by a fall, maximal at (9mm.Hg.) 6 hours which lasted for up to 62 hours. However in a group of twelve patients treated, by Ross & Drance, over a two week period with the 5% solution, only four showed a drop of 5 mm.Hg. after twice daily drug instillation at the end of that time. No change in outflow was seen. A tachycardia of up to 100 or 150 beats per minute was recorded in 50% of patients on one or more occasion. In addition marked irritation and redness occurred. The tachyphylaxis and severe side effects preclude the use of this drug, clinically, in open angle glaucoma.

SALBUTAMOL

This drug was studied by ourselves (Paterson & Paterson, 1971). The drug was used in a 4% solution. One single instillation lowered the IOP in all 16 patients studied. The extent of the fall varied with the height of the original IOP and from patient to patient. It became evident two hours after administration and reached a peak 8-10 hours later. The effect lasted up to 48 hours. Fig. 1 shows the result in a male patient aged 67 years. Fig. 2 shows the result on a patient, a man of 64 who received salbutamol at 9 a.m. on three successive days after initial control measurements. The results are represented as a range in the di-urnal variations of IOP on the control day -C, and three days of treatment to both eyes. The range of pressure on the second day of treatment was at lower limits than on the first day, although on the third day, there appeared to be some recovery in both eyes. Fig. 3 shows a comparision of range of di-urnal variations between 4% Salbutamol and 1% adrenaline. C is the control day, S is Salbutamol and A is adrenaline. On the basis of the concentrations used in this study, the fall in IOP induced by 4% Salbutamol, was equivalent to 1% adrenaline. However the longer term study which was carried out on nineteen patients with open angle glaucoma who were instructed to instill the drug daily proved disappointing. Over half of them developed an intolerable hyperaemia with irritation which led to the rejection of treatment. In addition one patient in five developed tachyphylaxis after as short a period as two weeks. No effect on the coefficient of aqueous outflow was demonstrated. No tachycardia occurred. Salbutamol is a β_2 agonist and therefore has little or no action on cardiac receptors. Thus what looked like a promising drug in theory, proved disappointing in practice and is of little clinical use in treating open angle glaucoma.

Investigation of the adrenergic agonists then shows that adrenaline 1% and nor adrenaline 4% are the most useful drugs on a long term basis.

Further research was directed towards potentiating their effects by creating a state of pharmacological denervation in the eye, with consequent super

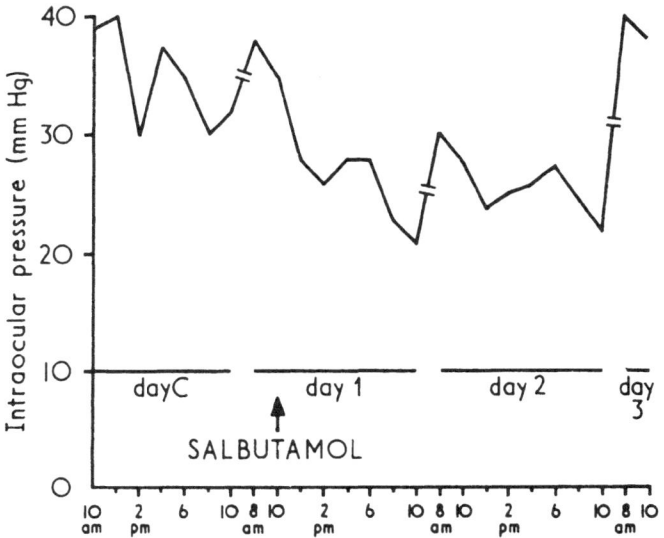

Fig. 1. The effect on IOP of a single instillation of salbutamol 4% eye drops.

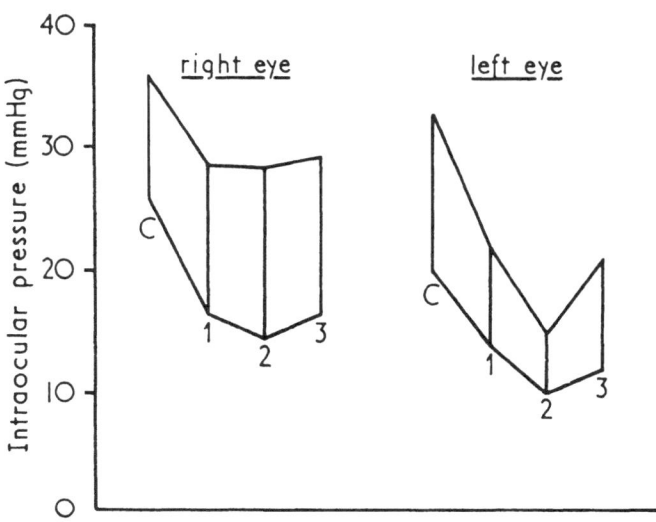

Fig. 2. See text

77

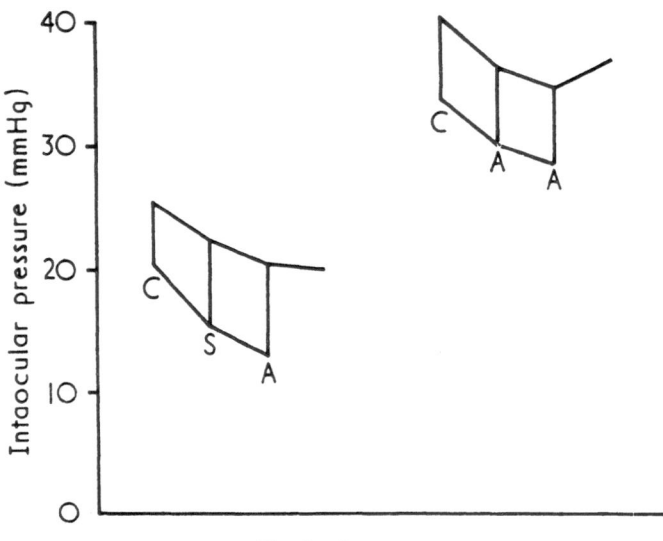

Fig. 3. See text.

sensitivity of the adrenergic receptors to either endogenous noradrenaline or exogenously administered adrenaline or noradrenaline.

PROTRIPTYLINE

Certain tricyclic anti-depressants prevent re uptake of adrenaline and nor adrenaline into the post ganglionic sympathetic neurones and thus potentiate the peripheral action of these catecholamines. Protriptyline was shown by Langham & Carmel (1968) to have ocular hypertensive and mydriatic effects, which were dependent on the presence of an intact sympathetic neuronal network in the eyes. Its ability to potentiate the ocular responses to exogenously administered noradrenaline has been demonstrated by Kitazawa & Langham 1968.

Kitazawa (1972) has used protripyline in the treatment of open angle glaucoma. He used the 0.5% solution which was instilled six times daily. In his study involving 24 patients, the base line pressure was 29.2 mm.Hg. ± 0.65 mm.Hg. and this dropped to 24.8 mm.Hg. ± 1.17 mm.Hg. at the end of one week. At the end of a month only 8 of the original series had pressures controlled under 20 mm.Hg. However 6 of these patients remained on the drug for one year. No topical side effects were noticed and only two complained of burning and stinging on the instillation of the drops. No systemic side effects were reported. Successful treatment with this preparation depends on the response of the patient. This has been shown to vary enormously and probably depends on basic sympathetic tone.

6-HYDROXY DOPAMINE

This has been used by Holland (1972) and Kitazawa, Nose & Horie (1975) to produce a chemical sympathectomy and thus potentiate the effect of adrenaline in the eye. Both groups of workers have used these drugs success-fully in the treatment of open angle glaucoma. The great disadvantage is that 6-Hydroxy dopamine itself is so unstable and becomes readily oxidised. It has to be freshly prepared just before administration to the patient. Because of poor penetration it has to be administered by Ionto-phoresis, subconjunctival injection or corneal bathing. A single application results in a chemical sympathectomy which lasts for up to 100 days. The potentiation to adrenaline is profound and allows concentrations of adrena-line as low as $(10^{-4})\%$ to be used to lower IOP. However as the days go by, the concentration of adrenaline has to be increased up to 2%, and when control can no longer be achieved at this concentration a further dose of 6-Hydroxy dopamine must be applied.

Following the application of 6-Hydroxy dopamine a transient lowering of IOP, due to the release of endogenous catecholamines occurs but is no longer present after three days. On its own, this drug is not useful for the treatment of open angle glaucoma. Holland demonstrated an average drop in pressure of 17 mm.Hg. or 85% more with 2% adrenaline in sympathec-tomized eyes compared with 6-Hydroxy dopamine untreated eyes in the same patient.

GUANETHIDINE

The drug guanethidine is a sympathetic post ganglionic blocking agent acting by preventing the release of nor adrenaline in response to nervous stimulation. It causes an initial depletion of nor adrenaline from the nerve fibre, blocks the neuronal release of the transmitter, and prevents re-uptake of catecholamines into neural stores.

Keates, Krishna & Leopold (1960) first reported its potential use in the treatment of open angle glaucoma. It is a pharmacological denervater of the eye and produces a ptosis and miosis similar to that seen in Horner's syn-drome.

The effect of 1, 2, 3, 4 and 5 percent solutions of guanethidine were examined by Paterson & Paterson (1971) in 9 patients (18 eyes) with ocular hypertension. After base line measurements, the subjects were phased for 24 hours after instillation of the drug at 10 a.m. They were then discharged with instructions to use the drug twice daily for one month. The five strengths of solution were tested by successively increasing the concentra-tions, two weeks being allowed to elapse between each investigation. The results are shown in Fig. 4 and Fig. 5 shows the increase in outflow which was demonstrated four hours after instillation of the first application of the drug, by tonography.

The average maximum fall in IOP 8 hours after a single instillation of guanethidine was -9.7 ± 1.1 mm.Hg. with the 3% solution and -7.3 ± 1.3 mm.Hg. with the 5% solution. This was reduced to $+1.00 \pm 1.00$mm.Hg. and -3.2 ± 1.4 mm.Hg. with the 3% and 5% solutions at the end of one month. Thus guanethidine produced an initial effective fall in intra-ocular pressure which is poorly maintained so that at the end of one month little hypotensive effect remains. This initial fall is almost certainly due to the release of endogenous catecholamines within the eye, and on

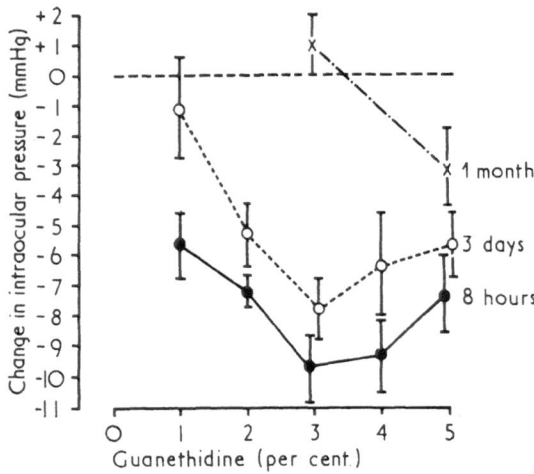

Fig. 4. The change in IOP after installation of different concentrations of guanethidine eye drops after 8 hours, 3 days and 1 month.

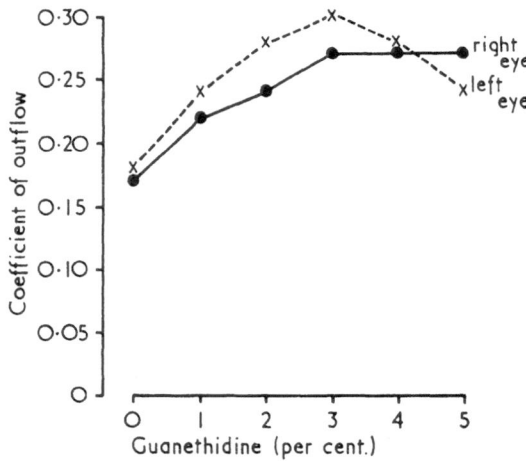

Fig. 5. The change in coefficient of outflow due to different percentages of guanethidine.

long term basis this drug is not useful in the treatment of ocular hypertension and open angle glaucoma. However when 5% guanethidine is combined with 1% adrenaline and both are instilled at twelve hourly intervals
with guanethidine preceeding the adrenaline by five minutes, the picture
changes. A fall in pressure of the order of 15mm.Hg. is achieved. Fig. 6
demonstrates this potentiation which is maintained on a long term basis.
The results of treating the first thirteen patients over a twelve month period
at our Glaucoma Unit in Moorfields Eye Hospital are shown in Fig. 7. This
therapy was introduced in 1970 and fifty-six patients were selected for a

study of treatment by this method. Forty-nine were suffering from open angle glaucoma or ocular hypertension, four patients had pigmentary glaucoma, two had the exfoliative syndrome and there was one case of congenital glaucoma. Some have remained controlled with IOP at 22mm.Hg. or less for more than five years now. Table 1 shows a more detailed analysis of the average pressure fall, in the different age groups, over a three year period.

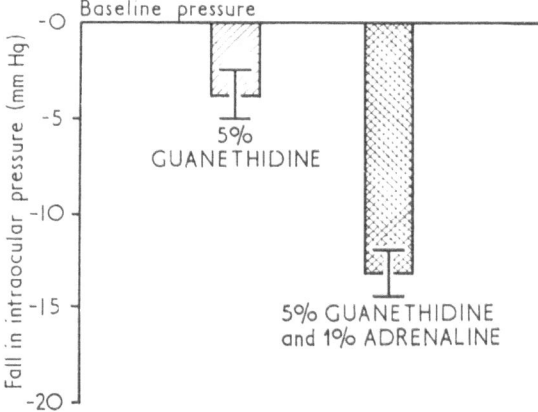

Fig. 6. Potentiation of adrenaline 1% eye-drops by guanethidine 5% eye-drops twice daily.

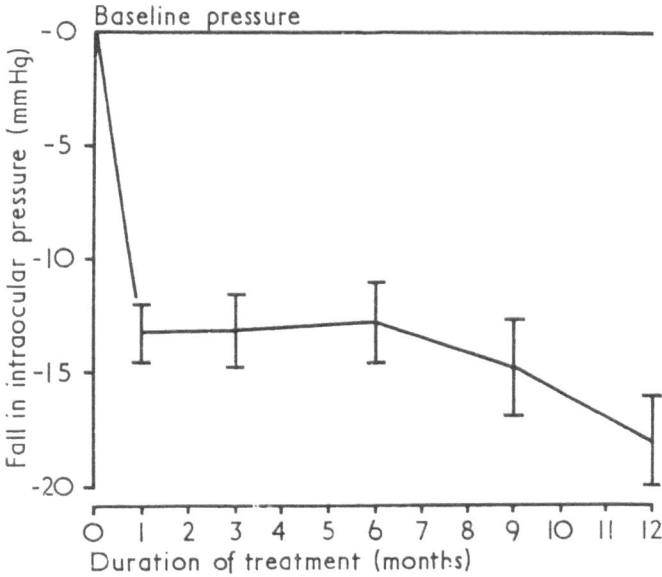

Fig. 7. Effect on IOP of a combination of adrenaline 1% and guanethidine 5% over a 12 month period.

TABLE 1. Response to treatment with 5% guanethidine and 1% adrenaline in the different age groups

No. of eyes	5	19	33	21	21	
Age groups	30 to 39	40 to 49	50 to 59	60 to 69	70 to 79	
Base line	48	32.8	32.1	33.7	31.3	mm Hg
1 week	22.8	21.0	19.8	21.1	19.8	
1 month	21.4	18.6	17.9	18.3	18.4	
6 month	20.0	19.2	18.0	19.2	18.2	
12 months	21.5	19.1	19.2	19.2	18.3	
24 months	22.0	19.2	19.2	19.3	19.0	
36 months	22.0	19.2	19.2	19.3	19.0	

TABLE 2. Number of eyes which developed allergy

	1/12	3/12	6/12	Total
No. of eyes	3	4	6	13

DURATION OF TREATMENT
(5% Guanethidine with 1% Adrenaline)

TABLE 3. Results (on 17 eyes controlled on 5% Guanethidine with 1% Adrenaline) of reducing the Adrenaline to 0.5%

MEAN BASE LINE PRESSURE			32.7 mm Hg	± 2.5
MEAN PRESSURE AFTER	2 YRS	5% G+A (1%)	18.5 mm Hg	± 0.9
MEAN PRESSURE AFTER	1/52	5% G+A (0.5%)	16.5 mm Hg	± 0.8
MEAN PRESSURE AFTER	1/12	5% G+A (0.5%)	17.6 mm Hg	± 0.8
MEAN PRESSURE AFTER	3/12	5% G+A (0.5%)	17.2 mm Hg	± 0.8
MEAN PRESSURE AFTER	6/12	5% G+A (0.5%)	17.5 mm Hg	± 0.9
MEAN FALL IN PRESSURE	6/12	5% G+A (1%)	−14 mm Hg	± 2
MEAN FALL IN PRESSURE	6/12	5% G+A (0.5%)	−15 mm Hg	± 2

The only significant finding was the much higher base line pressures in the youngest group which demonstrated a dramatic fall, maintained for three years in the five eyes in this group.

Of the original fifty-four patients, three died and one moved out of the area. In eight eyes control was not maintained. In thirteen eyes, seven patients, an intolerable allergy developed. This was characterized by swollen eyelids, conjunctival hyperaemia and punctate epitheliopathy of the cornea. Table 2 shows details of this complication with time intervals. Both the patients with the exfoliative syndome suffered the severe side effects and had to be withdrawn, along with the other five, from the study. Many patients suffer the hyperaemia, but prefer this to miosis. For this reason studies were undertaken to see if it would be possible to reduce the strength of the drug. Nine patients (seventeen eyes) who had been well controlled on the combination of guanethidine 5% and adrenaline 1% twice daily for more than two years were selected. Adrenaline 0.5% was substituted for the 1% solution and the results can be seen in table 3. In fact there was no significant difference in the hypotensive action between the 0.5% and 1% adrenaline with guanethidine and the hyperaemia was certainly reduced. The result of reducing the guanethidine to 3% was not quite so promising, and suggest that a tachyphylaxis develops after about three months in six patients studied. Tachyphylaxis was encountered rarely with the use of guanethidine 5% and adrenaline 1% as the long term results show.

This therapy provides a very useful non miotic regime for patients with open angle glaucoma and was particularly appreciated by the younger patients, including those with pigmentary glaucoma for whom it should probably be the treatment of choice. The older patients with lens opacities also preferred the non miotic therapy. Perhaps the therapy would prove even more efficient and the side effects be even further reduced if it could be administered in Ocusert form.

REFERENCES

Becker, B., Pettit, T.H. & Gay, A.J. Topical Epinephrine Therapy of Open-Angle Glaucoma. *Arch. Ophthal. (Chicago)* 66. 219 (1961).

Darier, A. Cited by H.S. Sugar. The Glaucomas (ref. 3) Kimpton London 1951. P. 179.

Holland, M.G., Treatment of glaucoma by chemical sympathectomy with 6-Hydroxydopamine. *Trans. Am. Acad. Ophthalmol. and Otol.* 76. 437. (1972)

Keates, E.V., Krishna, N. & Leopold, I.K. Effect of Guanethidine on intra-ocular pressure in glaucoma. Symposium on Guanethidine, Ciba, Memphis. (1960).

Kolker, A.E. & Becker, B., Epinephrine Maculopathy *Arch. Ophthal.* 79. 552. (1968).

Köllner *Munsch. Med. Wschr.* 65. 299. (1918).

Kitazawa, Y. Topical Adrenergic potentiators in Primary Open-Angle Glaucoma. *Am. J. Ophthalmol.* 74. 4. 588. (1972).

Kitazawa, Y., Nose, H. & Harie, T. Chemical sympathectomy with 6-Hydroxydopamine in the treatment of primary Open-Angle Glaucoma. *Am. J. Ophthalmol.* 79. 1. 98. (1975).

Langham, M. & Carmel, D. The action of protriptyline on adrenergic mechanisms in rabbit, primate and human eyes. *J. Pharmacol. Exp. Ther.* 163. 368. (1968).

Langham, M., Kitazawa, Y. & Hart, R.W.J. Adrenergic responses in the human eye. *J. Pharmacol. Exp. Ther.* 179. 47. (1971).

Paterson, G.D. & Paterson, G. Drug Therapy in Glaucoma. B.J.O. 56. 3. 288. 1972.

Paterson, G.D. & Paterson, G. A comparison of the ocular hypotensive actions of salbutamol and adrenaline in chronic simple glaucoma. *Postgrad. Med. J.* 47. 122. (1971).

Pollack, I.P. & Rossi, H. Norepinephrine in treatment of ocular hypertension and glaucoma. *Arch. Ophthal. (Chicago)* 93. 173. (1975).

Ross, A.R. & Drance, S.M. Effects of topically applied isoprotenenol in man. *Arch. Ophthal. (Chicago)* 83. 39. (1970).

Weekers, R. & Collignon-Brach, J. & Grieten, J. Contribution to the study of ocular hypotension caused by various sympathomimetic amines in Drug Mechanisms in Glaucoma. Churchill, London, 51. (1966).

Author's address:
c/o Moorfield Hospital
High Holborn
London WC1 V7AN
England

OCULAR HYPOTENSIVE EFFECT OF ATENOLOL 4% EYE DROPS IN GLAUCOMA

R.F. BRENKMAN

(Woerden)

INTRODUCTION

One of the most intriguing and daily recurring problems in the ophthalmological practice is glaucoma; for as we know every glaucoma patient has to face the fact their eye sight is failing, and that they may lose it altogether.

Our **knowledge** both as to how glaucoma is caused as to the progress of the various forms of glaucoma has largely increased, due to the work of many prominent researchers. But the **treatment** of these patients, and **that** is what we are daily concerned with, is often very difficult. Conservative therapy is given preference, as the success of surgical treatment is not always predictable, and surgical complications of a local and general kind may occur. Therefore surgical treatment is usually only considered as a last resort.

When prescribing local and if necessary general therapy for glaucoma, our aim is to reduce the IOP to such a level that either visual field loss is prevented, or the already existing visual field loss is prevented from spreading. In pursuing this, it has to be realised that the conventional medicins up to now, namely miotics, adrenergic drugs and carbonic anhydrase inhibitors have side effects. Therefore it's not unusual to find patients frequently either fail partly or wholly to carry out the prescribed treatment, or suffer inconvenient and in some cases harmful side effects. Furthermore in a considerable number of cases, no satisfactory pressure reduction can be achieved with these drugs even used in combination.

The ideal medical treatment is the one that is easy to apply, that has no side effects and brings about the required fall in IOP. The application of bêta receptor inhibitors, which have been especially developed in the field of cardiovascular diseases, appears to be a decisive step in the direction of this ideal treatment.

The first reports on the favourable effects obtained when these drugs were applied to the treatment of glaucoma, are based on findings after intravenous and oral administration of propranolol (Phillips, Howitt & Rowlands, 1967). These favourable results were confirmed in later publications (Coté & Drance, 1968), as was the suitability of local administration (Bucci, Pecori-Giraldi, Missiroli & Virno, 1968; Vale & Phillips, 1970; Vale, Gibbs & Phillips, 1972; Bietti, 1973).

Vale & Phillips (1973) published favourable results with Practolol eye drops on 8 patients. In 1974, on the annual meeting of the Dutch Ophthalmological Society, we reported on our own research concerning the pro-

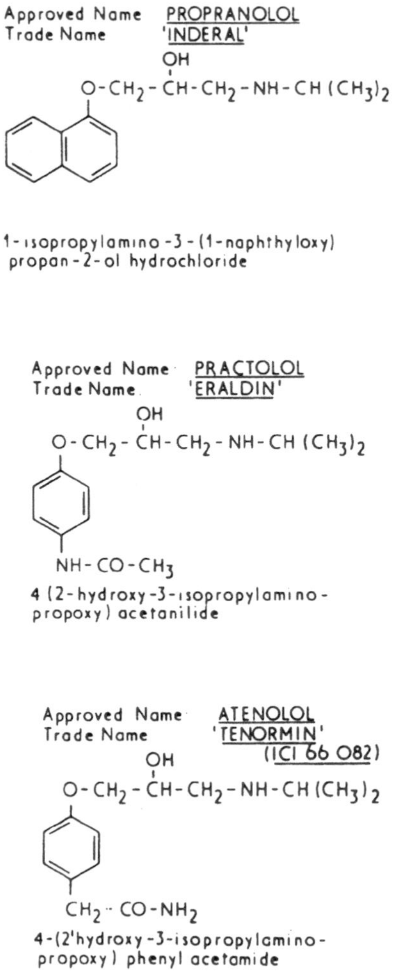
Approved Name PROPRANOLOL
Trade Name 'INDERAL'
OH
O-CH2-CH-CH2-NH-CH(CH3)2
1-isopropylamino-3-(1-naphthyloxy)
propan-2-ol hydrochloride
Approved Name PRACTOLOL
Trade Name 'ERALDIN'
OH
O-CH2-CH-CH2-NH-CH(CH3)2
NH-CO-CH3
4 (2-hydroxy-3-isopropylamino-
propoxy) acetanilide
Approved Name ATENOLOL
Trade Name 'TENORMIN'
(ICI 66 082)
OH
O-CH2-CH-CH2-NH-CH(CH3)2
CH2-CO-NH2
4-(2'hydroxy-3-isopropylamino-
propoxy) phenyl acetamide

Fig. 1. The structural formulae of propranolol, practolol and atenolol.

nounced IOP reducing effect of 10% Practolol eye drops in 38 glaucoma patients.

Stimulated by the favourable results published by Elliot et al. in 1975 with Atenolol (fig. 1), a new very specific bêta adrenergic blocker, which was orally administered, we started a research into the effect of Atenolol 4% eye drops. As we are of the opinion that, although systematic application may have its advantages when the patient is unable to administer the medicin locally, local treatment is the treatment of choice, since a high local concentration of the drug can be easily attained using this technique, without affecting the whole body.

MATERIAL AND METHODS; PLAN OF OUR RESEARCH
OBSERVATIONS AND DISCUSSION OF THE RESULTS

In this paper a description is given of the influence of the instillation of 4% Atenolol eye drops into the eyes of 11 glaucoma patients in whom glaucoma had not been previously detected (Table 1). The age of the patients varied from 50 up to 79; there were no special types of glaucoma involved.

TABLE 1. Material

11 patients (5 male, 6 female) in whom glaucoma had not previously been detected

age 50–79 years

gonioscopic classification:

wide angle	7
intermediate angle	2
narrow angle	2

(no special types of glaucoma)

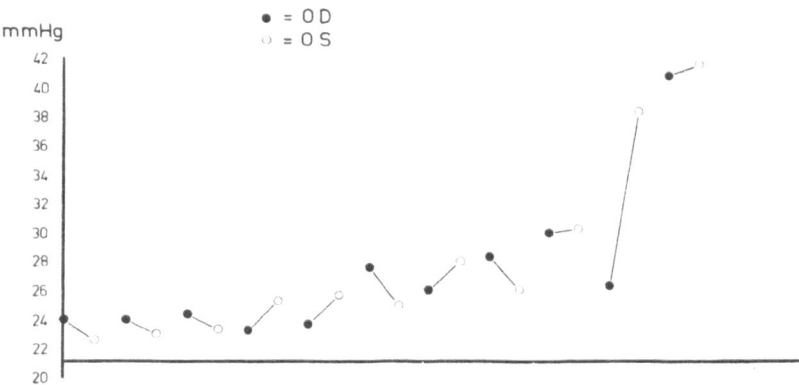

Fig. 2. Average IOP before instilling Atenolol (3 readings on different times).

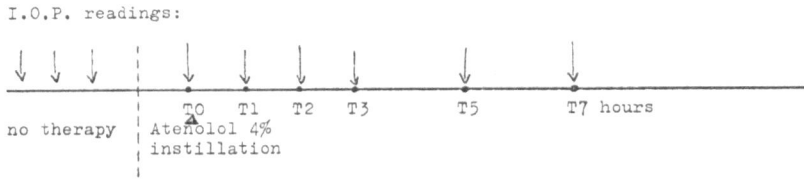

Fig. 3. Plan of our research.

87

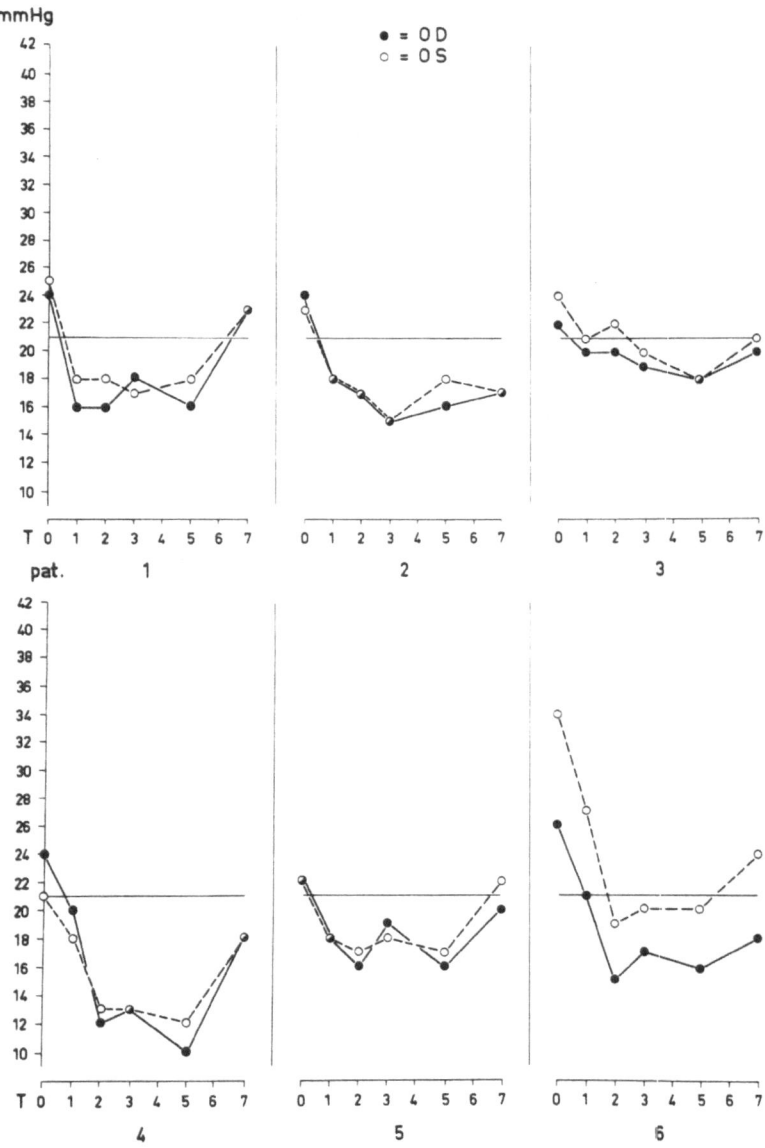

Fig. 4. The course of the fall in IOP after instillation of Atenolol 4% eyedrops.

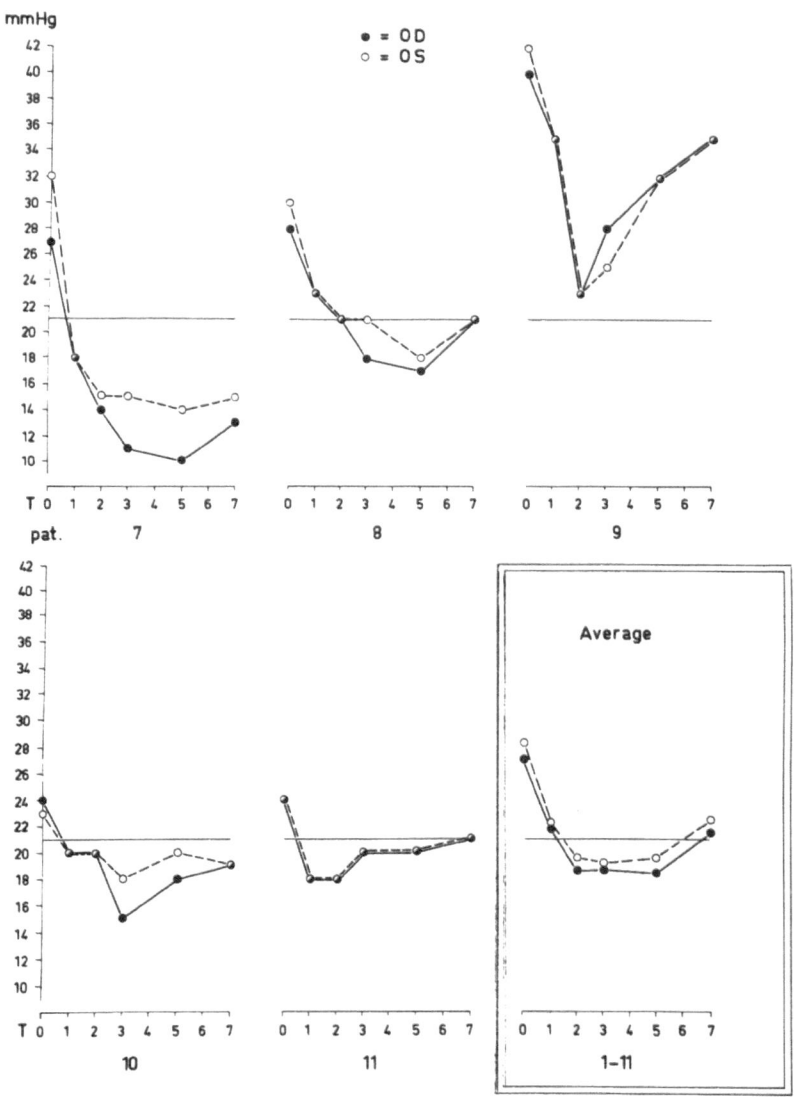

For our research the most important data gathered from our patients were: the ophthalmological case history including any concurrent systemic therapy, the fundus (optic disc), gonioscopy, perimetry, and the IOP. The IOP was invariably measured with the applanation tonometer.

The first thing we did was to measure the IOP in each patient three times on several days before the instillation of Atenolol eye drops.

In figure 2 you can see the average of the three readings of the right and the left eye before instilling Atenolol, arranged according to the height of the patients' initial IOP. In most patients we found this IOP to be between 22 and 30 mm Hg, in 3 patients more than 30 mm Hg, and in one patient even over 40 mm Hg.

Then we checked the effect of the instillation of two drops of 4% Atenolol eye drops in both eyes, during seven hours. For this we invariably measured at 9 o'clock in the morning the initial IOP, just before the instillation of the Atenolol eye drops (T O). Then we instilled two drops of Atenolol in both eyes and measured the IOP after 1, 2, 3, 5 and 7 hours (fig. 3).

In figure 4 the course of the IOP reduction after instilling Atenolol eye drops is graphically plotted for each single patient, and the average reduction for all 11 patients together is to be seen. In all patients we find a clear fall in IOP after instilling Atenolol eye drops. This pressure reducing effect appears to be more or less different for each individual patient, but remarkably similar for both eyes of one and the same patient; findings that are in agreement with our previous research into the effect of Practolol eye drops.

Generally we can already see a clear effect after 1 hour, that appears to have increased after 2 hours and which continues for five hours rather constantly. 7 hours after the instillation the IOP reducing effect appears to be decreasing. In general the effect appears to be more pronounced in those eyes in which the initial IOP was higher.

In figure 5 we have plotted the fall in IOP after 1, 2, 3, 5 and 7 hours for each individual patient, and the average of all patients together.

Especially when presenting the findings in this way, it appears that in some patients the IOP falls more strongly than in others, but that in one and the same patient both eyes generally react in a similar way.

The average fall in IOP of both eyes during seven hours after instilling Atenolol is to be seen on the bottom in the outlined figure. An average fall

TABLE 2. The average fall in IOP after instillation of atenolol 4% eye drops (patient 1–11)

After:	mm Hg fall:
1 hour	5.7
2	8.6
3	8.6
5	8.6
7	5.6

of more than 7 mm Hg was only found in eyes with an initial IOP of more than 26 mm Hg. An average fall of more than 10 mm Hg only in eyes with an initial IOP of 30 mm Hg and more.

In figure 6 we can see the course of the average fall in IOP of all 11 patients together during the seven-hour period, we observed the effect of Atenolol on the IOP. The greater part of the effect appears to be reached

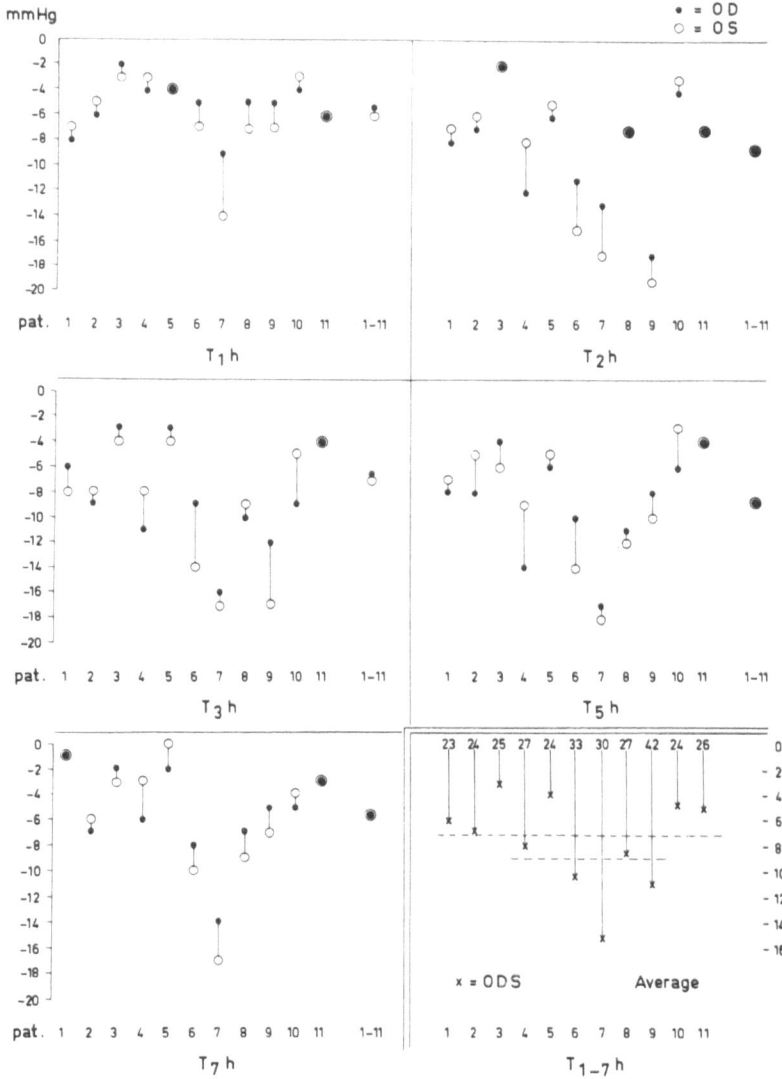

Fig. 5. The fall in IOP after instilling Atenolol 4% eye drops, after 1, 2, 3, 5 and 7 hours.

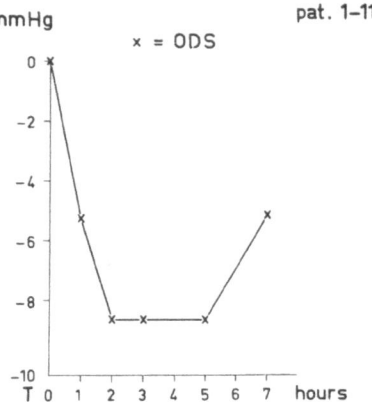

Fig. 6. The course of the average fall in IOP after instillation of Atenolol 4% eye drops (patients 1-11).

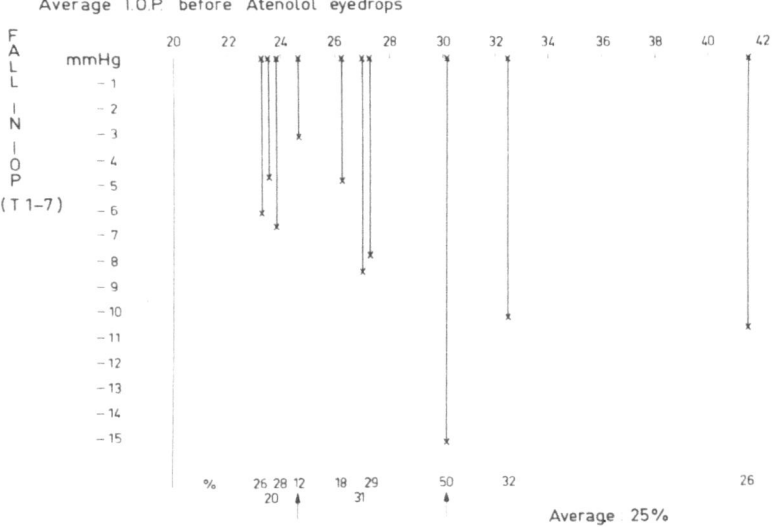

Fig. 7. The average fall in IOP after instillation of Atenolol 4% eye drops (T 1-7 hours) as related to the average of the three IOP readings before the instillation.

after 1 hour, namely 5,7 mm Hg. After this the IOP falls another 2,9 mm Hg, up to 8,6 mm Hg. Then the fall in IOP appears to be constant, that is 8,6 mm Hg, measured 2, 3 and 5 hours after the instillation. After 7 hours the average fall in IOP is less pronounced, although it is still 5,6 mm Hg (Table II).

In figure 7 we have plotted the average fall in IOP of both eyes during seven hours after the instillation of 4% Atenolol eye drops, related to the

TABLE 3. The advantages of atenolol (Tenormin ICI) eye drops

─ a pronounced hypotensive action
─ no influence on the size of the pupil
─ no blurring of the vision
─ no local irritation

average IOP of the three readings before we started our experiment, checking the influence of Atenolol eye drops in a 7-hour curve. The numbers at the bottom of the figure show the fall in IOP expressed as percentage of this initial IOP. In this way it is even more clear that although in general the number of mm Hg pressure reduction is greater as the case of glaucoma is more serious, there is a rather constant relation between the number of mm Hg pressure reduction and the height of the initial eye pressure before medication, namely a pressure reduction of 25% calculated with regard to this initial pressure. The arrows indicate that one patient showed only half, one patient twice the average reduction of IOP.

DISCUSSION

From our findings we can conclude that Atenolol eye drops have a pronounced IOP reducing effect, and that generally spoken we may expect that the IOP in a glaucoma patient will decrease about 25% expressed as percentage of his initial IOP. One patient may react far less strongly or far stronger.

The fact that these eye drops have no influence on the size of the pupil, do not cause any blurring of the vision nor any irritation when instilled into the eyes, are important extra advantages (Table III).

Another advantage lies in the fact that in the cases where local application is impossible, it is possible to perform systemic administration with the same effect on the IOP.

Through the application of bêta receptor inhibitors for non ophthalmic reasons by specialists for internal diseases and neurologists in their treatment of hypertension and tremors, it is not inconceivable that glaucoma patients get a 'regulated' IOP (Hagedoorn & Tjoa, 1974). In this respect it is also conceivable that in a number of potential sufferers from glaucoma the IOP does not even get the chance of rising to injurious degrees.

To get an impression about the pressure reducing effect in the long run, and in combination with the conventional medication in those cases where this fails to bring about the required fall in IOP, a follow up study is undoubtedly necessary. Our experience with a number of patients who have now been using Practolol eye drops for more than two years, is encouraging in this respect.

To maintain a normal level of IOP, turned out to be an extremely complex mechanism on which the autonomic sympathetic system has a great influence. As both stimulation and inhibition of adrenergic receptors can cause IOP reduction, it appears that alpha, bêta-1 and bêta-2 receptors have their own influence which is partly independent of one another. Both stimulation of the one kind of receptors and blockade of the other kind may cause a similar effect, so that the apparently conflicting situation arises that as well sympathomimetical as sympatholytical drugs can cause intraocular pressure reduction.

Among other Musini (Musini, Fabbri, Bergamaschi & Mandelli, 1971), Takats (Takats, Svilvssy & Kerek, 1972), Vale (Vale & Phillips, 1973) and Bietti (Bietti et al., 1973) have given a dissertation on the way in which bêta-receptor blocking drugs work pressure reducing; but for the time being the mechanism does not stand out very clear.

We have the strong impression that in the future bêta-adrenergig-blocking agents will turn out to be a welcome addition to the Medical Therapy in Glaucoma.

REFERENCES

Phillips, C.I., Howitt, G. & Rowlands, D.J. *Brit. J. Ophthal.*, 51, 222. (1967).

Bucci, M.G., Missiroli, A., Pecori-Giraldi, J. & Virno, M. *Boll. Ocul.*, 47, 51. (1968).

Coté, G. & Drance, S.M., *Canad. J. Ophthal.*, 3, 207,. (1968).

Vale, J., Gibbs, A.C.C. & Phillips, C.I. *Brit. J. Ophthal.*, 56, 770. (1972).

Vale, J. & Phillips, C.I. *Exp. Eye Res.* 9, 82. (1970).

Bietti, G.B. Klin. Mbl. Augenheilk., 162, 281 (1973).

Vale, J. & Phillips, C.I. (1973) *Brit. J. Ophthal.*, 57, 210.

Hagedoorn, A. & Tjoa, S.T. *The Lancet*, april 20, page 733. (1974).

Musini, A., Fabbri, B., Bergamaschi, M. & Mandelli, V. *Am. J. Ophthal.*, 72, 4. (1971).

Takats, I., Szilvassy, I & Kerek, A. *Albrecht von Graefes Arch. Klin. Exp. Ophthalmol.*, 185, 331 (1972).

Elliot, M.J., Cullen, P.M. & Phillips, C.I. *Brit. J. Opthal.*, 59, 296 (1975).

Author's address:
Vossenschanslaan 142
Woerden
The Netherlands

USE OF OXPRENOLOL EYE DROPS IN GLAUCOMA PATIENTS

J.S. STILMA

(Amsterdam)

The increasing frequency of cardiac diseases has initiated an at least equal increase of beta adrenergic blocking drugs. It has been demonstrated that propanolol has the ability to reduce the intraocular pressure when given orally, by retrobulbar injection, or when applied as eye drops. (Coté 1968, El-Shewy 1969, Öhrström 1973, Vale et al. 1972)

Another beta-blocking drug, practolol, has also this property but after the description of the adverse effects by P. Wright (1975) its use is limited in cardiology as well as ophthalmology. (Hagedoorn 1974, Vale & Phillips 1973, Wettrel 1976)

Oxprenolol, also a beta-blocker was selected in this trial after two observations:

1. Two glaucoma patients with cardiac disease showed a 10 mm reduction of their intraocular pressure after the administration of oxprenolol 40 mg three times daily. Withdrawel of this drug was followed by an increase of the intraocular pressure.

2. Ocular side effects of oxprenolol has not been described before our investigation started. (CIBA 1975, Fucella 1969, Meyler 1971)

MATERIAL AND METHODS

After the kind permission of Ciba-Geigy the oxprenolol eye drops were prepared in our hospital pharmacy. The formulation used was:

R/ oxprenolol 200 mg, solutio acidi borici 8 ml, solutio boracis conservans 2 ml.

The patients selected for trial were seven male and four female, with an age range of 32-74 years. All patients had evident or suspected glaucoma simplex.

Previous treatment has been stopped on the day before the investigation started.

After the first applanation readings at $9.^{00}$ one drop oxprenolol 2% was applied in the conjunctival sac of one eye.

The other eye served as a control.

RESULTS

The fellow eye showed usually an increase of the intraocular pressure.

The eyes with the oxprenolol drops showed a significant reduction of the

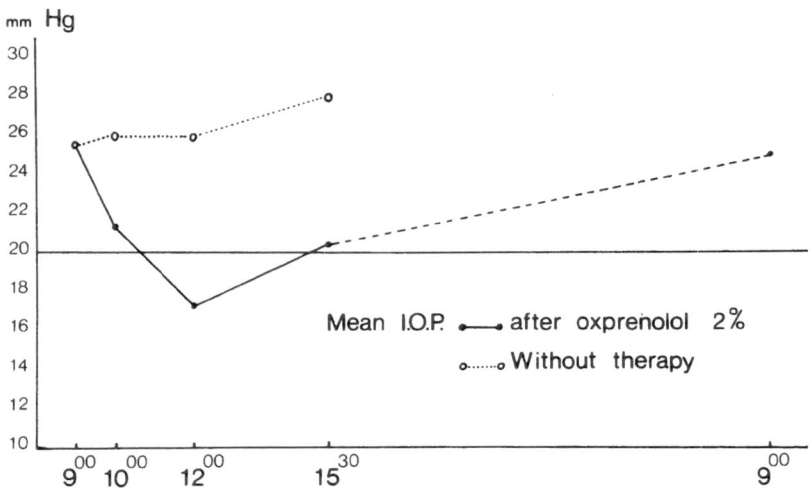

Fig. 1. Mean intraocular pressure in 11 patients
without therapy . . . .
after oxprenolol 2% ————

intraocular pressure. In one patient the ocular tension dropped from 40 untill 20mm.

The mean intraocular pressure at 9^{00} was 25,5 mm.

After one drop oxprenolol the readings at 10^{00}-12^{00} and 15^{30} were in succession 21,5-16,7 and 20,2 mm.

In four patients we were able to establish that after 24 hours the intraocular pressure was on the same initial level again. (See fig. 1).

Besides the lowering of the intraocular pressure oxprenolol has the advantage to maintain the full range of accomodation. In one case A scan ultrasonography was performed before and after the administration of oxprenolol eye drops.

The depth of the anterior chamber as well as the lens thickness have not changed.

Unfortunately two disadvantages appeared during this investigation.

First, a marked corneal epitheliopathy with some blurring of vision developed in the last two patients. Within one day the cornea has completely recovered without therapy. Second, during the trial two reports about ocular side effects were published. (Holt 1975, Knapp 1975)

This effects were similar with the oculomucocutaneous syndrome as described for practolol.

FINAL REMARKS

Oxprenolol eye drops 2% can produce a significant reduction of the intraocular pressure without serious disturbance of the pupillary size and the accomodation. This experience may serve as a stimulation for further developments of medical therapy in glaucoma.

Because of the side effects of this 2% formulation, it is not the most suitable one for glaucoma patients. But, maybe in the future there is another beta-blocking drug which is more convenient to glaucoma patients. (Elliot et al. 1975)

ACKNOWLEDGEMENT

I am grateful to Prof. C.M.J. Velzeboer and Prof. A. Hagedoorn for help and kindness. I should also like to thank Dr. Tjoa for coöperation. F.A. Boom, pharmacist, did take care of the preparation and conservation of the eye drops.

REFERENCES

Ciba-Geigy, letter for information (1975).

Coté, G., Drance, S.M. The effect of propanolol on human intraocular pressure. *Canad. J. Ophthalm.* 3, 207-212 (1968).

Elliot, M.J., Cullen, P.M., Phillips C.I. Ocular hypotensive effects of atenolol (Tenormin I.C.I.) *Brit. J. Ophthalmol.* 59, 296-300. (1975)

El-Shewy, T.M., Amin, E. Effect of beta-adrenergic blockade with propanolol on the intraocular pressure. *Bull. Soc. Ophthalm. Egypt* 62, 95-102 (1969).

Fucella, L.M., Imhof, P. Experience with a new beta-blocking agent (Trasicor[R]) in the management of cardiac arrhytmias. *Pharm. Clin. (Berlin)* 1, 123-13 (1969).

Hagedoorn, A., Tjoa, S.T. Practolol in the control of ocular tension. *Lancet* 1, 733. Letter (1974).

Heilman, K. Medikamentöse Glaukomtherapie (Stuttgart, 1974).

Holt, P.J.A., Waddington, E. Short report. *Brit. med. J.* 2, 539-540 (1975).

Knapp, M.S., Galloway, N.R. *Brit. Med. J.* 2, 557. Letter (1975).

Meyler, F. Side effects of drugs. Volume VII (1969-1971).

Öhrström, A. Clinical experience with propanolol in the treatment of glaucoma. *Acta Ophthalm.* 51, 639-644 (1973).

Vale, J., Gibbs, A.C.C., Phillips, C.I. Topical propanolol and ocular tension in the human. *Brit. J. Ophthalm.* 56, 770-775 (1972).

Vale, J., Phillips, C.I. Practolol (Eraldine) eye drops as an ocular hypotensive agent. *Brit. J. Ophthalm.* 57, 210-214 (1973).

Wettrell, K., Wilke, K., Pandolfi, M. Effect of beta-adrenergic agonists and antagonists on repeated tonometry and episcleral venous pressure. European Congress of Ophthalmology, Hamburg (1976).

Wright, P., Untoward effects associated with practolol administration. *Brit. Med. J.* 1, 595-598 (1975).

Author's address:
Department of Ophthalmology
Free University Hospital
1105 De Boelelaan
Amsterdam
The Netherlands

CRITERIA FOR THE INITIATION OF TREATMENT IN PATIENTS WITH SUSPECTED GLAUCOMA

P. GRAHAM

(Cardiff)

It is my task to introduce the subject of when, and in whom to start active treatment for chronic glaucoma.

There is, I think, only one absolutely unequivocal indication, and that is the eye with established, repeatable glaucomatous visual field change allied to an IOP which is above or at the upper end of the so-called 'normal' range. It is, in practice, in this state that many chronic glaucoma patients present, and there is no problem about the decision on whether to start treatment, though the most desirable form of therapy may be arguable. Today however, increasing awareness of the possibility of prevention of field loss and the widespread use of tonometry as a routine component of the ophthalmic examination frequently faces the ophthalmologist with the problem of deciding whether or not prophylactic treatment is justifiable or necessary in the absence of any perimetric abnormality.

The art − for it is not yet a science − of making this decision lies in the apprecation of two facts. Firstly, so-called 'ocular hypertensive' − that is those whose IOP are higher than could reasonably occur in a population with normally distributed IOP − progress only at a very slow rate to the development of field defect. The rate appears so low, a maximum of about 4 per 1000 per year having been estimated, that it is highly probably that many will never succumb in their lifetime. Secondly, all prophylactic therapy causes rather than relieves symptoms. What we are doing, therefore, is trying to balance the risk of permanent damage to vision through the withholding of active treatment against the disadvantages of taking a asymptomatic patient − probably happy until we saw him − and giving him iatrogenic symptoms which may make him miserable, or at least reduce the quality of his life. (Fig. 1.).

At one end of the spectrum of decision we have the young or middle-aged healthy patient, with no cardiovascular disease, no family history of glaucoma and normal discs who is found to have a 'raised' IOP. Here the risk is almost directly proportional to the level of IOP and *even at fairly high levels it is a low risk*. (Fig. 2). In such a younger patient, still economically active, the side effects of miotic therapy are both severe and disabling. We can afford to watch, tailoring the frequency of observation to the level of his IOP. At the other end we have the elderly patient with suspicious looking discs but no field defect, diabetic, with a history of cardiovascular disease, and having a parent or sib with chronic glaucoma. Even a moderate

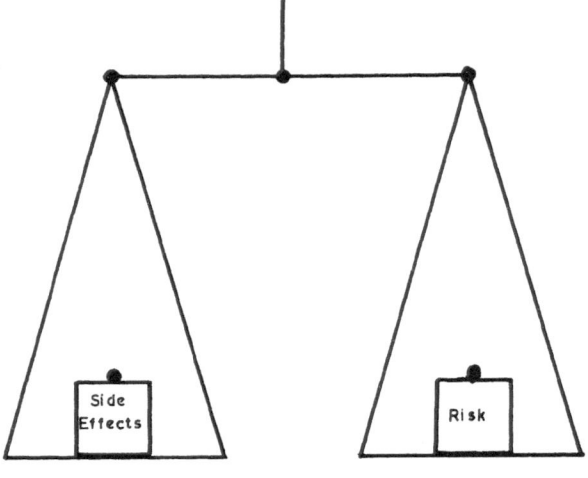

Fig. 1.

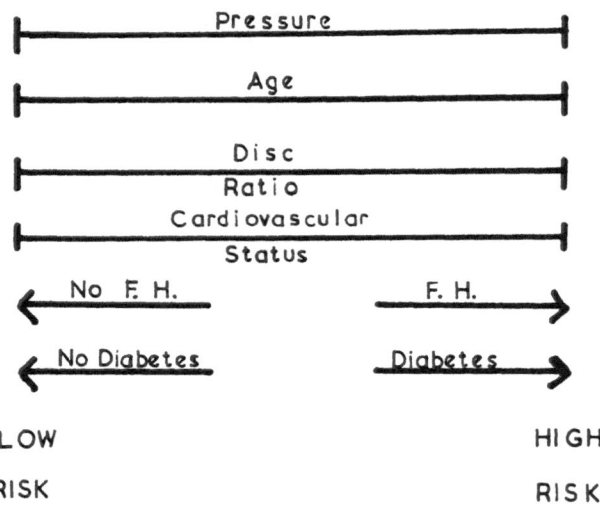

Fig. 2. Risk factors in decision-making.

elevation of IOP probably carries a high risk in such a patient and vigorous efforts to reduce it are justifiable even side effects occur.

Let us examine more carefully this balancing process. To achieve it we require an assessment, as precise as possible, on the one hand of the probability that a glaucomatous field defect will appear, and on the other of the side effects of the miotic or miotic and adrenaline therapy which we would be most likely to prescribe for prophylaxis.

There is ample evidence by now that the probability of the development of visual loss correlates with IOP. Though the evidence for this is very good, it must however, be made clear that the correlation, though undoubtedly significant, is far from close. There is no level of IOP at which field loss is impossible, and very high levels must be reached before it can be considered inevitable. For practical purposes there is a large range of IOP over which other criteria must be used to decide the extent of risk and therefore the desirability of treatment. Only at fairly high levels of IOP — I think many of us use 30 mm. Hg. (applanation) though we may well be over cautious — does the level of IOP override other considerations. If at these intermediate levels, we are to make a valid assessment of the risk, we must not only consider the IOP, but also try and estimate the probable susceptibility of the eye to that level of IOP. Failure to do so, and the use of the simple approach that 'mean pressure plus one, or two standard deviations = treatment' will condemn many unfortunate patients to a pointless endurance of the disadvantages and discomforts of the miotic life. We can therefore subdivide the risk side of the balance into two components: — pressure; and susceptibility to pressure. The higher the latter, the lower the acceptable IOP before risk outweighs side effects.

There is no problem about the assessment of IOP. The difficulty lies in the fact that the precision of the measurement does not mean that we can easily define what is 'normal' IOP for any individual, for normal IOP is that at which no damage occurs, and we have already noted that though IOP and damage are correlated, the relationship is not a close one. What, then, do we know about the factors which determine this variable susceptibility?

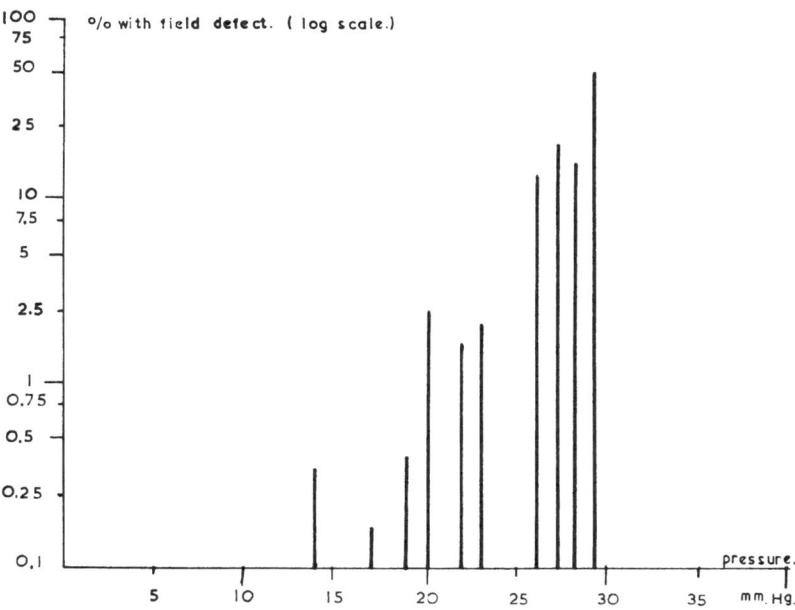

Fig. 3. Rising prevalence of field defect with rising pressure.

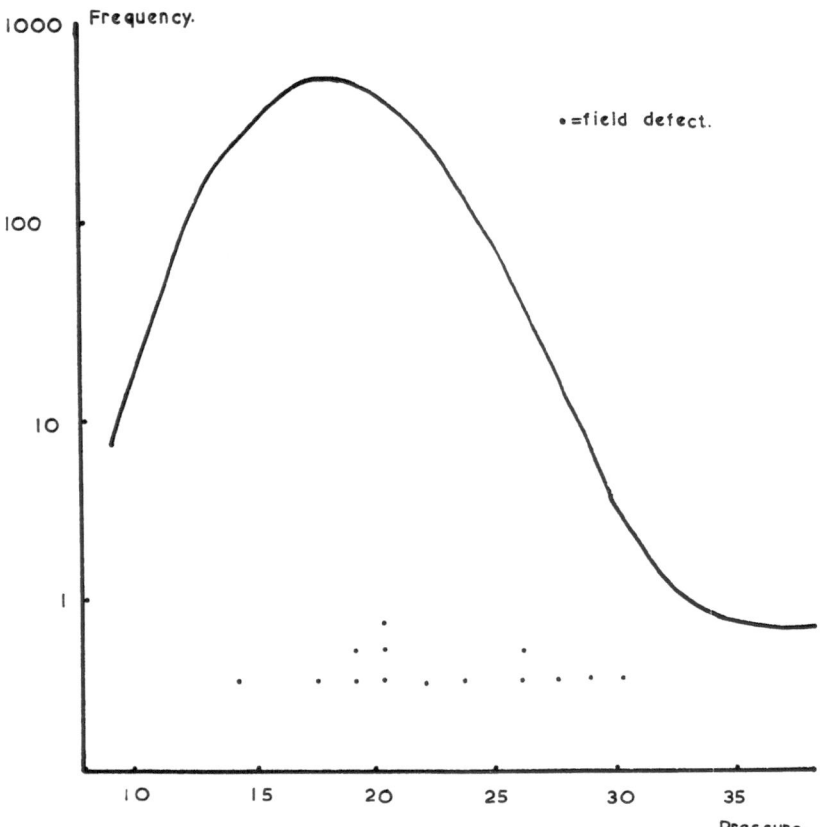

Fig. 4 Correlation between field defect and pressure is not close. Defects can occur at statistically 'normal' pressures.

In terms of patho-physiology, there is fairly good evidence that one major factor is the state of the circulation at a critical point in the supply to the optic nerve just within the eye . This portion appears to be very susceptible even to moderate elevations of IOP, and a low perfusion pressure at this point may mediate increased susceptibility to the effects of raised IOP or even determine damage at levels of IOP which in relation to the rest of the population must be considered quite normal.

Though various attempts have been made to access the IOP at this critical point, or the level of IOP at which it becomes inadequate, none is yet sufficiently developed or evaluated to have general clinical application. Nor do tonography or the long-established provocative test such as water-drinking or the priscol test assist us, for essentially they measure determinants *of*, or liability *of*, IOP not susceptibilty *to* IOP, and do not take us any further than IOP itself. We must for the present rely much more indirectly on the patient's general cardiovascular status and his age. The poorer the former and the greater the latter (and in this respect we should consider not chronological age, but biological age as assessed from appearance and behaviour) the more likely it seems that perfusion pressure will be poor and the disc more susceptible to damage. The incidence of glaucoma increases with advancing age, and the increase seems to be more than can be accounted for simply by the known upward drift of IOP with age.

We also know that glaucoma has a notable hereditary tendency. The pattern of inheritance is such as to suggest that both IOP and the incidence of glaucoma are to a considerable extent determined in a multigenetic man-

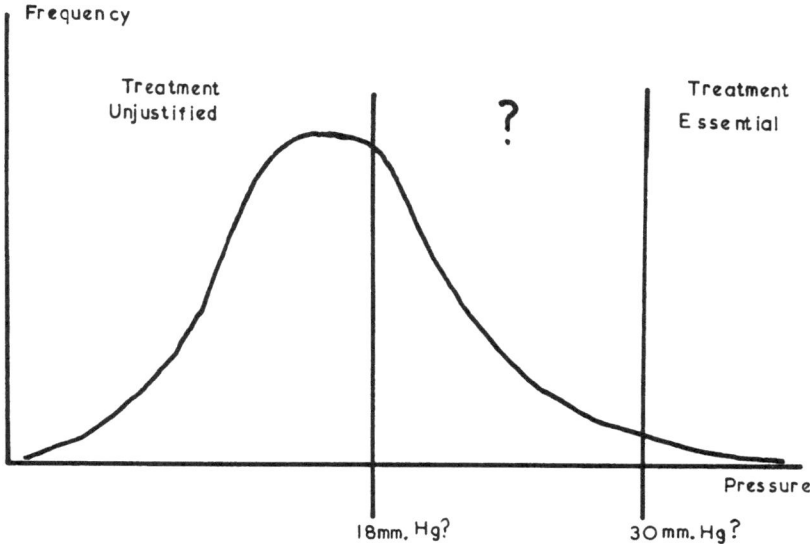

Fig. 5. In the zone of uncertainty pressure alone is insufficient for therapeutic decision-making.

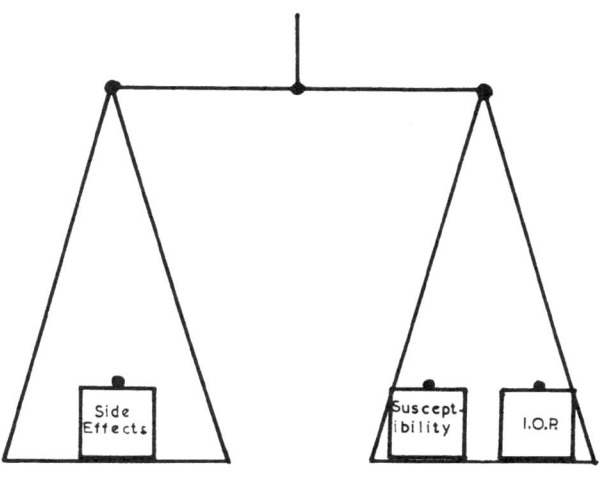

Fig. 6.

103

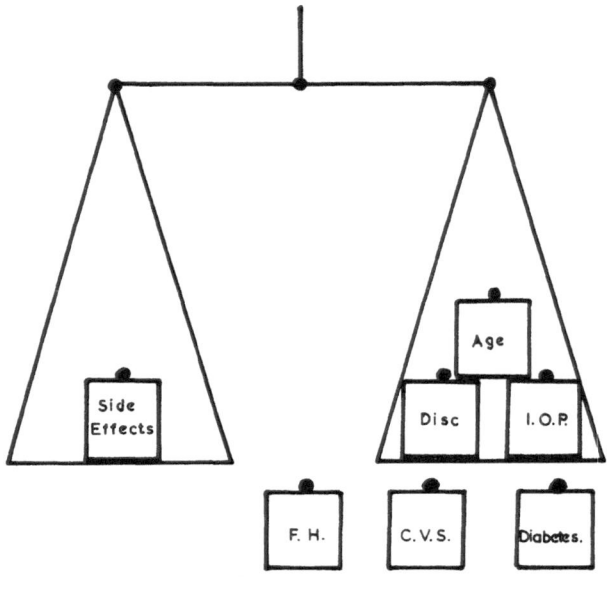

Fig. 7.

ner — that is, several genes are involved, so that the classical Mendelian pattern is not evident. While some of the increased incidence of glaucoma in children and sibs of known cases may be due to the genetic determination of higher IOP levels in these groups, the increase — for glaucoma may be up to fifteen times more common in such persons than in those with no family history — seems greater than can be attributed to raised pressure alone. Untill and unless it can be proven otherwise, it seems sensible to regard the patient with a family history of chronic glaucoma as more susceptible to elevation of IOP as well as more likely to exhibit the phenomenon.

In relation to general diseases other than the cardiovascular group, there is a demonstrable association between diabetes mellitus and glaucoma, which occur together more frequently than is likely by chance. Whether this is a reflection of the increased incidence of cardiovascular disease or due to other factors is interesting, but not relevant to our present purpose. We can make use of the known association and regard diabetics with increased suspicion.

Finally in the assessment of susceptibility comes a more positive criterion, and that is the appearance of the disc. Though glaucomatous field defects do occur in association with normal-looking discs, this is uncommon and the vast majority are associated with discs which look pathological to the experienced eye. Thus the cup disc ratio is a useful objective guide, for the appearance of the disk may change before any functional defect can be detected. Other things being equal, the higher the cup-disc ratio, the more probable the development of field change, whereas the pink, normal looking disc with a small cup of less than one third of the disc diameter is much less vulnerable, or at any rate less likely in the short or medium term to be associated with the development of a field defect. Vertical ovality or irregularity in the shape of the cup and assymmetry between the two eyes are also of help in assessment, although very much less so than the cup-disc ratio.

With the exception of IOP and the cup-disc ratio, none of the factors I have discussed is easily quantifiable. The assessment we make is in the nature of an intelligent and informed guess. This does not mean that it is not worth the effort, and it is certainly better than reliance on tension measurement alone − the 'magic-number' approach, in which pressure in excess of some hypothetical upper limit of 'normal' are automatically treated.

Turning now to other side of scales, we require an assessment of the side-effects and disadvantages of therapy for the individual patient. To this I would now add that one must, before embarking on a policy of long-term medication, be sure that it is achieving its' immediate aim of reducing IOP. Here the problem is simpler. There will be cases in which the risk is assessed so low that the correct policy is clearly to watch, or even to dismiss, and others in whom the probability of damage is so high that serious disadvantages would have to be clearly demonstrated before a watching brief could be accepted. In between, there are many in whom the ballance is fairly even. The obvious course to adopt in this case is so ascertain at least the short-term disadvantages of treatment by practical trial. It must be clearly understood, not only by the patient, but by the ophthalmologist, that this initiation of treatment is an experiment to discover its' suitability for this one individual. There are two objectives: 1). To find if the treat-

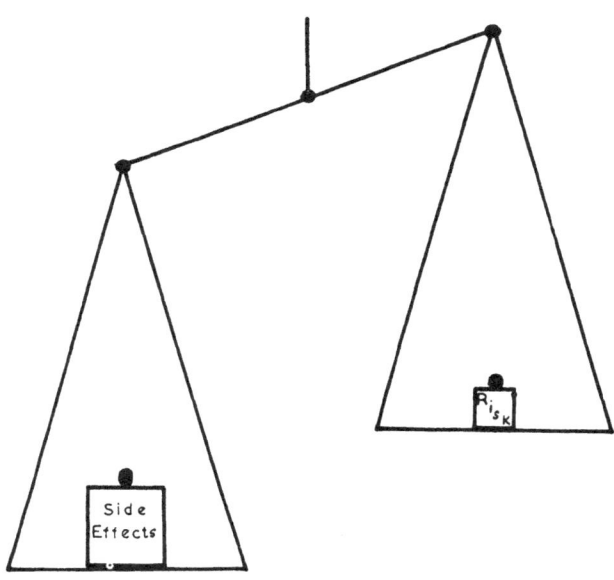

Fig. 8.

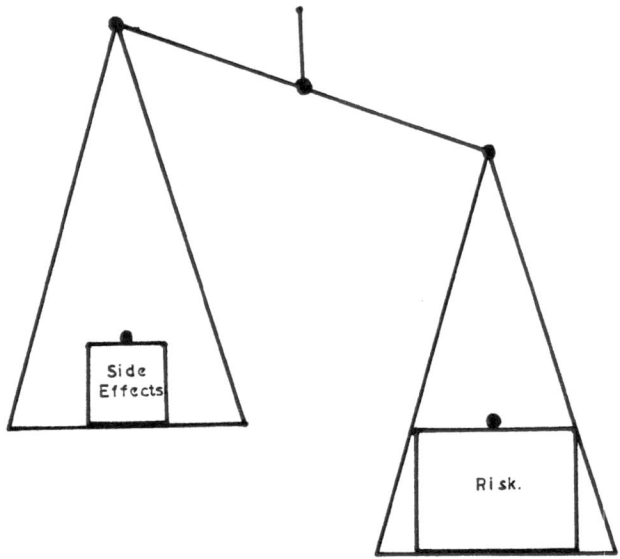

Fig. 9.

ment is acceptable to the patient. 2). To demonstrate that the treatment *does reduce IOP*, for it seems very improbable that medication which does not do so serves any useful purpose. The former is very largely subjective, though the effects of miotics on refraction and acuity can be directly measured. The latter requires some care, and is often overlooked, for it is not uncommon on reviewing the records of glaucoma clinics to find that miotic therapy has been started after one or two visits, a small fall in IOP has been observed, and treatment thereafter continued in the assumption that thiss fall was the effect of the treatment. May be; but this is not always so, for the IOP is quite often higher on the first two or three visits, and the latter fall may have little or nothing to do with the treatment. I have frequently taken such patients off all treatment and observed no significant rise in IOP over long periods, so that one is forced to conclude that their period on treatment was probably valueless.

This error can be avoided by two simple procedures. Firstly, treatment of these patients is never urgent; we can therefore take time to establish the behaviour of the untreated IOP before starting the trial of treatment. The initial fall, if any, will be discounted, and we will have some idea of the extent to which the patient's IOP varies naturally. It may, of course, be desirable to observe the diurnal variation rather than to rely on a series of widely spaced single estimations. Secondly, in many cases the IOP in the two eyes is very similar or identical; if the therapy is used initially in one eye only, the demonstration that a consistent difference appears between the treated and untreated eyes is convincing evidence of therapeutic efficacy.

This balancing procedure will in many cases produce a fairly clear bias in

106

the mind of the ophthalmologist in favour of observation or active treatment. There will still, however, remain a residue in whom the virtues and vices of treatment are fairly evenly balanced. In those patients, who from my original premise have no field defect, I would suggest that it is quite legitimate to adopt an attitude of bias toward observation, provided that it can be effectively carried out. The critical feature of the observation process is the observation of the disc and visual field as well as attention to a rising trend in IOP. Observable change in the disc or the development of the typical early scotomata in the Bjerrum area − which, it should be noted, may be reversible − alters the balance and requires that a reassessment be made.

Having arrived at a decision that treatment is both justifiable and that it does reduce IOP, what should be the criterion of effectiveness? I would suggest that, although the appearance of a field defect must of course be noted, this event is a sign not that treatment is about to fail but that it has already done so, and that perimetry as a means of assessing the adequacy of control, in cases where the risk of field loss is considered high, is unsatisfactory. We must therefore rely on the IOP. The adoption of a set level below which IOP *must* be reduced is beset by the same dangers as those already discussed in relation to the starting of treatment. The desirable level depends on the assessment of susceptibility, and what for one is safe is dangerous for another. I would suggest that in assessing the adequacy of treatment, we should pay much more attention to the reduction in pressure as a proportion of the untreated IOPP than to its' absolute level. A reduction from 40 mm. Hg. to 25 mm. Hg. in a patient with normal looking discs should, in theory, provide a large margin of safety, and to insist on reducing the IOP further to 20 mm. Hg. or less is probably unwise and undesirable, whereas in the older subject in whom the disc is highly suspicious and whose untreated IOP is 30 mm. Hg., reduction to 25 mm. Hg. would be a fall of only 17%, against almost 40% in the first case. Perhaps in the case it would be more realistic to aim at a similar reduction, and try to get the IOP down not to 20 mm. Hg. but to 18 mm. or below. It would be of great interest to relate the success of glaucoma therapy in preventing the progression or appearance of field defect to the percentage reduction in IOP rather than to the absolute level achieved by treatment. I suspect the correlation would be better, but there are no really satisfactory data as yet to prove this point. It seems a reasonable hypothesis, however, and one on which it is reasonable to act unless it be proved false.

Author's address:
76 Cathedral Road
Cardiff CF1 9LN
Great Britain

SOME ASPECTS OF THE MANAGEMENT OF GLAUCOMA PATIENTS

E.L. GREVE

(Amsterdam)

I. EXAMINATION OF THE PATIENT

Definition

Glaucoma is the disease in which the IOP is too high for continued mainte-
nance of visual function. If one accepts the vascular theory, glaucoma is that
disease in which the perfusion pressure of the capillaries of the optic disc is
insufficient for maintaining function of the nerve fibre bundles at the optic
disc. The two main points of concern are the IOP on the one hand and the
local blood pressure in the capillaries of the optic disc on the other hand.

Patients which are found to have a raised IOP are called *glaucoma sus-
pects*. The raised IOP is not the only reason for suspicion as will be illus-
trated later on. If in addition to the raised IOP functional damage is found,
we speak about *established glaucoma*. The term ocular hypotension is frequently used in the literature, but we prefer the term glaucoma suspect.

Intra-Ocular Pressure IOP

What is normal IOP? From population studies we have learned that the
frequency distribution of normal IOP is between 9 mm and 21 mm. 2.5% of
the normal population have IOP above 21 mm. 0.15% of the normal population have IOP above 24 mm. The population surveys however showed that
the distribution of IOP was not a Gaussian one. Specially in the older age
groups the percentage of IOP above 21 mm is higher. The distribution is
skewed at the upper end. Thus individuals without glaucoma can have IOP
above 21 mm (mean + 2 x standard deviation). We have also learned from
population surveys that the occurrence of established glaucoma is much
lower than the occurrence of a raised IOP. This occurrence is far below 1%.
This means that the raised IOP is not equivalent with glaucomatous damage
or future glaucomatous damage.

IOP and probability of damage

What is the relation between IOP and functional or anatomical damage? In
other words what is the probability that a certain IOP will cause functional
damage. This question can be divided in two questions: *How high* can the

IOP be in the individual without causing functional damage and *how long* can an individual stand a certain raised IOP? Goldmann has introduced the term 'critical IOP'. This is the upper limit of the non-damaging IOP. The ideal situation would be if we knew this critical IOP of the individual patient. Follow-up studies of untreated patients with raised IOP are scarce. The few studies that exist with a follow-up of 5 or 10 years show that the percentage of patients with raised IOP that develop visual field defects is very low. This illustrates the fact that glaucoma is a chronic disease. A much longer follow-up of about 15 to 20 years is probably necessary to provide more information about the period between the rise of IOP and functional damage.

In the individual without visual defects the critical IOP is not known. The only thing we know is that this patients IOP is above the statistically normal IOP. We do not know when and at what level this IOP will cause functional damage.

Variability of IOP

Although the IOP is probably the best measurable parameter in glaucoma, it is by no means an invariable parameter. The IOP measurements depend on ocular rigidity, on squeesing of the eyelids, on erect or supine position of the patient, on the time of the day, on the age of the patient, on the mental stress, on the use of alcoholic or non-alcoholic liquids, and on sports or other physical exercise. Although the applanation tonometer is a fairly accurate instrument the variation of measurements between observers can still be fairly large. A difference of 5 mm between measurements of two observers is not uncommon, though they usually do not surpass 2 to 3 mm. There is no such thing as *the* IOP of a patient but *there is the range or diurnal* variation* of IOP of a certain patient. The normal diurnal (and nocturnal) varation is 3.7 ± 1.8 mm. In the glaucomatous patient this variation is much larger being 11.0 ± 5.7 mm (Drance; 1960).

The *type* of IOP variation is different in each individual. But it is usually typical and constant in the untreated glaucoma patient. Several types of 24-hour-variation have been described (Fig. 1). Important is the differentiation in a night type were the IOP peak is at night and a day type were the IOP occurs during the day. Often the peak IOP of the day type is in the early morning hours (7-9 hrs) but this peak may also occur at noon or late in the afternoon. Fortunately the day-type variation is by far the most frequent (about half of all types; *see table 1*). The night type makes up only 10% of the glaucoma patients.

Apart from the night-type and the day-type, a varying type, a flat-type and a peak-type have been described. The varying type has two or more peaks. The peak-type has irregular high peaks probably due to intermittent angle closure in patients with narrow angles. It can only be concluded that the individual IOP curve has to be measured in each glaucoma patient.

---

* The adjective diurnal comes originally from the latin word 'dies', which means day. Diurnal can best be used as opposite to nocturnal, a diurnal curve then is an IOP day curve. Diurnal ànd nocturnal IOP measurements constitute a 24-hour curve.

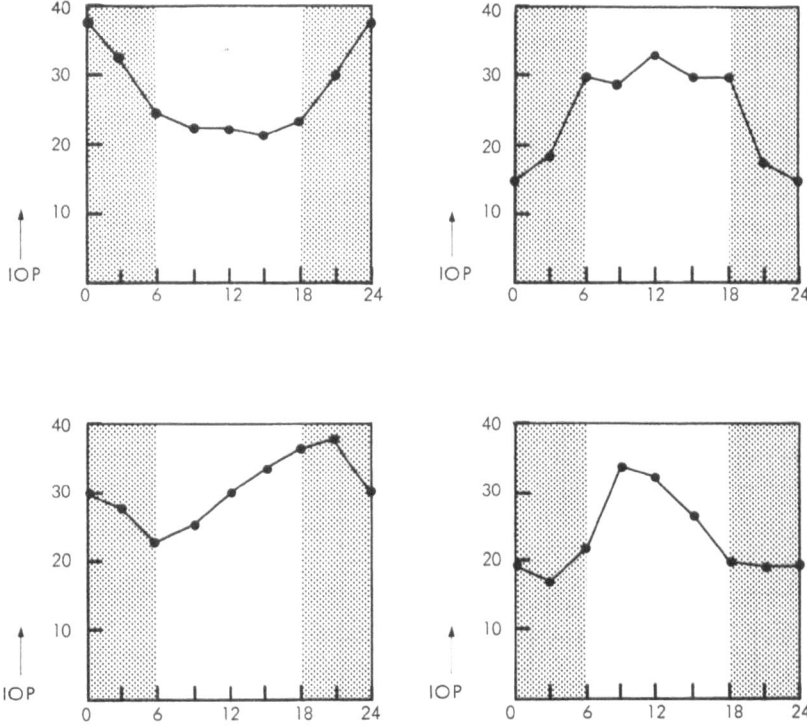

Fig. 1. Exaggerated demonstration of the four types of IOP curves. left upper: night type; right upper: day type; left lower: evening type; right lower: morning type.

TABLE 1. Frequency of different types of diurnal and nocturnal variation expressed as a percentage (after Hager; 1958)

	♂	♀	all
day type	66.7	36.7	49.3
night type	5.4	12.8	9.7
flat type	12.0	22.9	18.3
varying type	13.0	23.8	19.3
peak type	2.4	3.7	3.4

Usually a diurnal IOP curve will be sufficient for the practical management of a glaucoma patient. It is an essential criterium for the evaluation of the effect of therapy. If unexpected deterioration of the visual field occurs a nocturnal IOP curve has to be made.

Indicators of future damage

Since the problem of the glaucoma suspect was fully realized, investigators have tried to find tests that indicate the probability of future damage in a glaucoma suspect. However no such indicator has been found up till now. *Tonography tests, water drinking tests, cortico-steroid tests only tell us something about the IOP and not about the probability of functional damage.*

So the major problem in glaucoma remains still to predict the development of functional damage in the individual patient because there are no indications that will allow the identification of the susceptibility of an individual to develop the disease (see also Wilensky & Podos; 1975).

Suspicion of the presence of glaucoma

Not withstanding the lack of knowledge about the progression of events leading from raised IOP to field loss, the measurement of the IOP is still an important part of the detection of possible glaucoma patients.

Suspicion however of the presence of glaucoma can be aroused not only by the *level* of the IOP but also by the diurnal variations and differences between measurements of the left and the right eye. A right-left difference of more than 4 mm. is unusual. A rise of IOP after cortico-steroid drops is a reason for suspicion.

Apart from the IOP the presence of a nerve fibre bundle defect and/or 'pathological' cupping needs further investigation. A family history of glaucoma necessitates further examination, as well as some of the following findings: high myopia; central vene occlusion; pigment dispersion; pseudo-exfoliation; diabetes.

Visual field examination

Visual field examination is one of the most important examinations for the glaucoma patient. It is not the purpose of this symposium to describe extensively the best procedures for visual field examination. Some important facts will be mentioned here shortly. If the ophthalmologist has found a raised IOP he needs to know whether his patient is a glaucoma suspect or an established glaucoma. As we will see later on the management of these two stages of the disease is different.

It is necessary to divide visual field examination in a *detection phase* and an *assessment phase*.

The detection phase aims at accurate discovering of the presence of a visual field defect. For the *detection phase* the type of early defects in glaucoma have to be known and the area where they manifest themselves. The smallest size and least intensity of a glaucomatous defect determine the sensitivity necessary for the detection phase. At present in our clinic the detection phase consists of examination of the 30° radius visual field by means of multiple stimulus static perimetry (visual field analyzer) and examination of the peripheral visual field by means of kinetic perimetry (Fig. 2). This detection procedure will detect most of the early defects in glaucoma. For more details the reader is referred to Greve; 1973, Greve and Verduin; 1976, Greve; 1977. The detection phase is not difficult to carry out. If in the detection phase no defect is found, the patient remains a glaucoma suspect and the ophthalmologist has no immediate means of establishing whether his particular range of IOP is above or below the critical IOP.

A different situation exists once a defect has been found. We than proceed with the *assessment phase* in which the topography and intensity of a defect are accurately plotted. The established glaucoma patient needs more extensive therapy than the glaucoma suspect and secondly the presence of a visual field defect makes it possible to establish over a period of time whether a given IOP range is damaging or not. In other words the careful follow-up of visual field defects makes it possible to get an impression of the critical IOP. *This difference between a glaucoma suspect and a patient with established glaucoma with regard to critical IOP is stressed.* The assessment phase unfortunately is much more elaborate and requires more time, skill, ex-

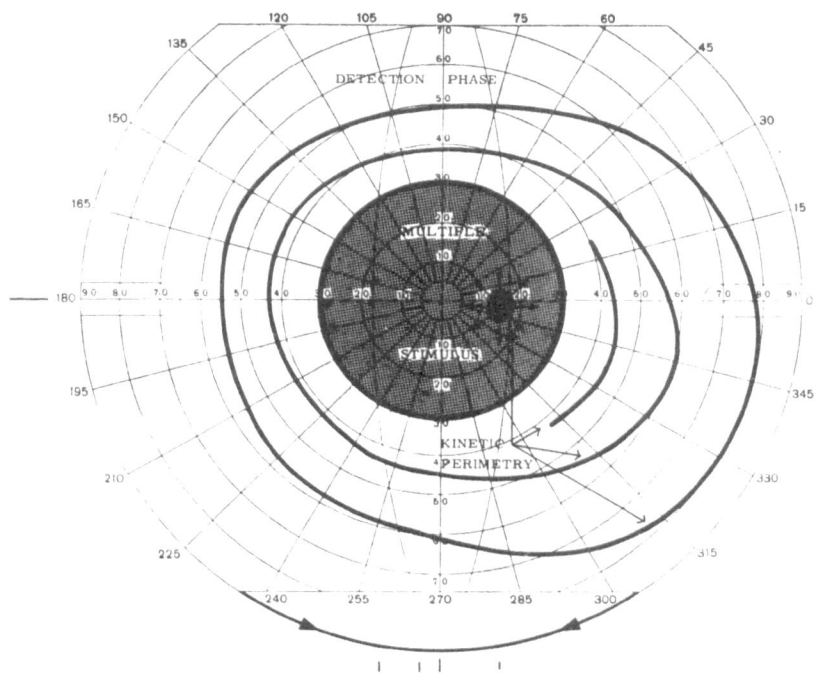

Fig. 2. Detection procedure; multiple stimulus static perimetry (visual field analyzer) in the central 30° field and kinetic perimetry for the periphery and the blind spot.

perience, dedication, knowledge and apparatus than the detection phase. It is in the assessment phase that many examinations of glaucoma patients often fail and therefore ophthalmologists tend to rely rather an IOP and optic disc than on the very essence: visual functional damage. The assessment phase can best be carried out by the well-known but scarely practiced procedure of combined kinetic and static perimetry.

In a symposium on medical therapy it should not be forgotten that *important therapeutic decisions are to be made on the basis of the assessment phase of visual field examination.*

The Optic Disc

The evaluation of the optic disc goes hand in hand with visual field examination where the *detection* of damage is concerned. In the *later stages* of glaucoma a good correlation exists between cupping and visual field. If this correlation is absent one should be very suspicious of the presence of other diseases than glaucoma alone. In the *early stages* of glaucoma however one can find visual field defects without recognisable pathological cupping and vice versa. The correlation is by no means as clear as in the later stages. This is the conclusion of an investigation of glaucoma patients without defects or with early glaucomatous defects that we recently carried out in our glaucoma department (Greve & Verduin, 1976). The consequences of this conclusion are that one can not rely or either of the two methods *alone*. A suspicious disc asks for carefull control and so do early visual field defects. In our opinion detection of damage by evaluation of the disc only is no service to the patient.

Once a visual field defect is present the evaluation of progression depends on visual field examination. Progression of damage can not be established with sufficient accuracy by ophthalmoscopy. Hemorrhages of the optic disc may be a bad prognostic symptom (Drance, personal comm).

Gonioscopy

No patient should be treated without having a good gonioscopic examination. The differentiation between a wide angle and a narrow angle is essential for the interpretation of therapeutic effects. In a wide angle the diagnosis of glaucoma may be easier if one finds subtle signs of developmental malformations in the chamber angle. Such signs are anterior insertion of the iris, a number of iris processes attaching to the spur or the trabecular meshwork, and these two signs in combination with a pronounced Schwalbes line. It is to be remembered that chronic simple glaucoma may exist with a narrow angle.

If one finds a narrow angle with a raised IOP then there are two possibilities: either there is a narrow angle with a chronic simple glaucoma, or there is a narrow angle with goniosynechiae. The presence of goniosynechiae indicates that there have been episodes of intermittent angle closure. In the latter case there is a good chance that a serious chronic narrow angle glaucoma will develop with high peaks of IOP.

If one finds a narrow angle with a normal IOP the presence of goniosynechiae may indicate that the angle is occludable. If in the case of a narrow angle and a normal IOP there are no goniosynechiae we want to know whether this angle is capable of angle-closure. We then have to decide whether a prophylactic peripheral iridectomy is necessary or not. This is a difficult decision that requires experience in gonioscopy of narrow angles.

It should not be forgotten that the development of goniosynechiae in a narrow angle means the change from a narrow angle glaucoma patient that might be satisfactory controlled with a peripheral iridectomy to a chronic narrow angle patient that needs more than a peripheral iridectomy. In chronic narrow angle glaucoma there is always the risk of malignant glaucoma after a filtrating operation. Therefore the gonioscopic findings are essential for the therapeutic decisions in glaucoma.

Full first examination

For us a full examination includes the following:
1. Eye.
   a) general examination including visual acuity.
   b) IOP diurnal curve (if necessary nocturnal measurements, or comparative erect-supine measurements).
   c) gonioscopy.
   d) examination of disc and the rest of the fundus (diabetes, vessels, lattice degeneration etc.).
   e) photograph of the disc.
   f) visual field.
   g) if necessary ophthalmodynamometry or tonography.
2. General health.
   a) history (bleeding, diabetes, periph. vascular disease).
   b) systemic blood pressure.
   c) heart function.
   d) peripheral vascular disease.
   e) blood (diabetes, anaemia, clotting mechanism).
   f) general medical therapy (e.g. β-blockers).

If there are any doubts about the general health of the patient he should be referred for full internal medical examination. This is not only of importance for establishing the risk factors (e.g. a low blood pressure) but also for establishing the risk of anti-glaucomatous therapy (e.g. effect of adrenaline on the heart; diamox and kidney stones).

Motivation of the patient

Before medical therapy is started the patient is entitled to a full information about the nature of the disease. Once the ophthalmologist knows what type of glaucoma the patient has and in what stage of the disease the patient is, he can explain to the patient why or why not medical therapy is started. A patient with motivation will take his drugs much better than the patient who does not know what is going on. In general the recognition of long range goals is poor. The diagnosis of glaucoma does not help the patient what so ever. Only if the need for treatment has been effectively explained to the patients satisfaction and he has received adequate instructions, the patient will cooperate. The most significant correlation between proper use of medication and a demonstrable characteristic of the patient is his knowledge of the nature of the disease. There is no correlation between proper medication used and the following variables: age, sex, race, income, occupation, apparent intelligence or fear for blindness. Patients with considerable visual field defects are usually more reliable in taking their medications.

II. THERAPEUTIC CONSIDERATIONS

Purpose of therapy

It is the physicians role to determine the minimum quantity of drugs necessary to achieve his therapeutic objective. Such an approach often involves a greater amount of physician time than seems practical in a busy schedule and paradoxically traps the physician into seeking security in 'maximum medical therapy'. The therapeutic objective in glaucoma is to prevent loss of visual function or further loss of visual function by lowering IOP or increasing the circulatory conditions at the optic disc. As we have seen the relation between IOP and visual function is not a direct one so that not only measurements of IOP serve as a control for the effectiveness of therapy, but also and mostly so the examination of the visual field. Any discussion of medical therapy in glaucoma is necessarily a generalizing discussion. For the right application of therapy one should realize that it is necessary to individualize. Each patient has his individual type of glaucoma and his individual reaction on medical therapy. Each drug has apart from the desired effect on IOP the undesired side effects on the eye or on other parts of the body.

A schematic representation of therapeutic considerations in chronic simple glaucoma is given in fig. 3. Using this figure as a guideline we will discuss the medical management of the glaucoma patient.

Beginning of therapy. (see also Graham in this volume)

The beginning of therapy in a patient with established glaucoma is no problem because it is proven that the range of IOP of this patient is damaging and needs reduction.

In the case of a glaucoma suspect however we deal with probability and not with certainty of future damage. We do not want to trouble the patient with unnecessary medication and we want to save him the side-effects of therapy if possible. This means that we have to consider in every individual case of a glaucoma suspect whether it is worthwhile to start therapy.

Waiting for visual field defects

It has been suggested to wait with medical therapy till a visual field defect has developed. This then presents the ophthalmologist and the patient with an understandable reason for the beginning of medical therapy. The ideal case would be that medical therapy could be started in a stage when the

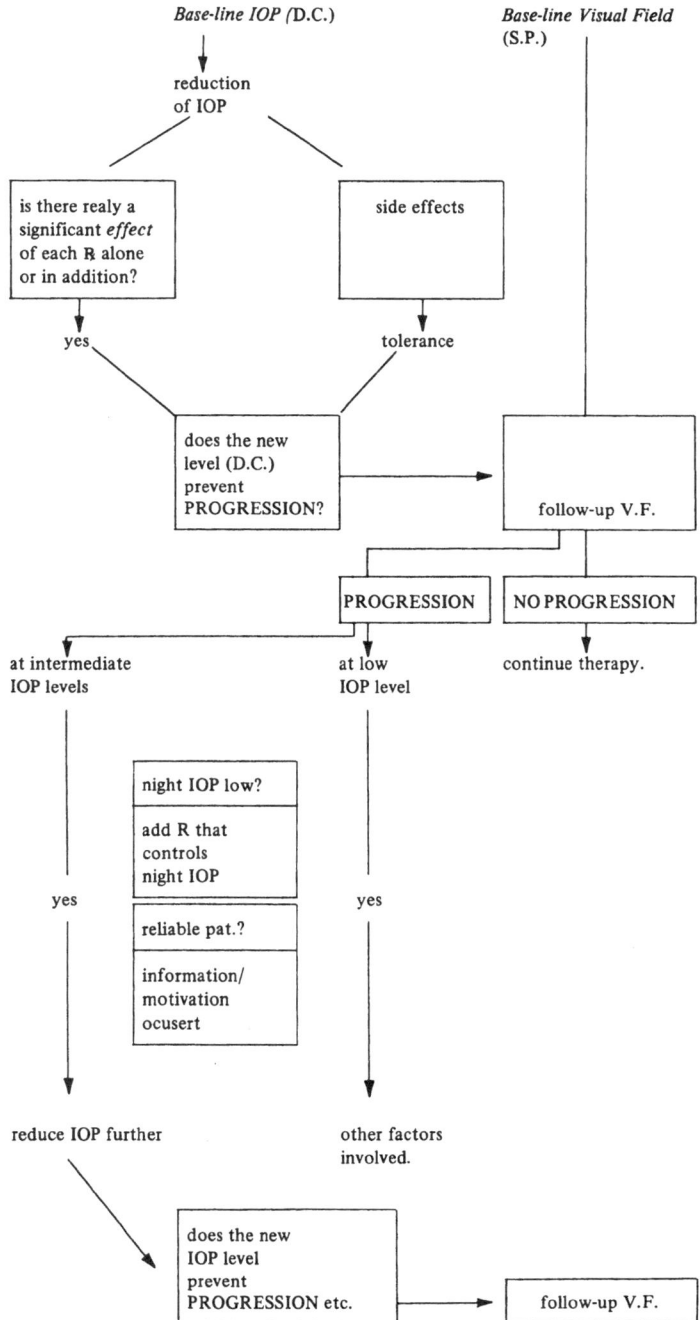

Fig. 3 Schematic representation of therapeutic considerations in chronic simple glaucoma; D.C. = diurnal curve; S.P. = static perimetry.

visual field defects are still reversible. It is however very difficult to defend this point of view in extremo, because the natural history of development of visual field defects still has many unknown features. It is not known whether visual field defects are always reversible in an early stage of their development and if so whether we are able to find these types of defects. Nor is it known whether the first visual field defects are always small and relative or whether suddenly large parts of the visual field can be lost.

Arbitrary level of IOP

Because of these uncertainties and because it is our task to prevent damage we have agreed upon an arbitrary level of IOP, above which medical therapy has to be started anyway. Let it be stressed that this arbitrary level depends on many other factors in addition to IOP. The decision whether to begin therapy or not depends on a combination of the IOP level and the risk factors. Most of us agree that therapy has to be started if some of the IOP measurements are over 30 mm. Goldmann feels that every IOP that is regularly higher than 25 mm should be treated.

The risk factors that have to be considered for the beginning of medical therapy in a glaucoma suspect are: 1. appearance of the optic disc; 2. family history of glaucoma; 3. systemic blood pressure; 4. obstructive vascular disease (carotic artery, small vessels); 5. heart disease; 6. diabetes; 7. age of the patient.

Other well-known factors that are included in therapeutic decisions are the presence of a cataract, the mentality and understanding of the patient, the profession of the patient and the possibility of the patient or his relations to administer the medical therapy.

Evaluation of therapeutic effects

Let us return to fig 3. Before we can start therapy we need two important data. First we need a baseline IOP diurnal curve (d.c.) without therapy and second we need a baseline visual field, preferably with accurate static perimetric measurements. All further evaluations of the effect of therapy will be based upon comparison with these baseline data. The IOP diurnal curve is indispensable for any appreciation of the real effect of medical therapy. One or two scattered IOP measurements will not serve for this purpose. The IOP diurnal curve gives information about the highest IOP and also about the variation of IOP during the day. With this curve as a guideline we start medical therapy. We wish to determine the individual sensitivity of the patient to a certain therapeutic agent and for each agent separately and in addition to the others. We want to get the best effect and the least side-effects with the lowest concentration and the lowest frequency of application. It seems so easy to establish that a certain therapeutic agent has a significant effect on IOP. In practice however it requires many comparative measurements to exclude that we are not dealing with normal variations of IOP. For instance if our first measurement *without* therapy is at 12 o'clock as indicated in fig. 4 and our second measurement *with* therapy is at 6 o'clock, we get a false impression of effectiveness of therapy. The reduction of IOP of approximately 5 mm is not due to the medical therapy but due to the normal variation of the IOP as shown in the diurnal curve. We find it very convenient to start the medical therapy in one eye and to use the other eye as a control. The reaction of both eyes of one patient to IOP reduction is usually equal. Sometimes the IOP of the untreated eye is reduced to some extent by local therapy of the other eye. The control of the therapeutic effect of the treated eye can be done by an IOP diurnal curve or by measurements of the IOP at the time where the IOP without therapy is highest. The ideal situation exists of course if the therapeutic effect of each agent is measured in a series of IOP diurnal curves. This however is very time consuming. If several agents have been tested and one is satisfied with the therapeutic response and if there are no untolerable side -effects, it is advisable to repeat the IOP diurnal curve in both eyes with therapy. If these last measurements are again satisfactory we can leave the patient on this regime for a considerable time.

What we have done so far is to reduce the IOP. From fig. 3 we can see that the next question is: does the new IOP level prevent progression of visual field defects? This is the one and only essential question. To answer this question we have to do a follow-up visual field examination. Generally spoken we repeat the visual field after one year. There may be reasons for a more frequent control. If there is no progression of the visual field we can continue the same therapy. If there is progression of the visual field with therapy there are several possibilities. If we have managed to reduce the IOP to low levels it could be that the patient still has IOP peaks at night. If our measurements with therapy show a low IOP level it may be that the patient

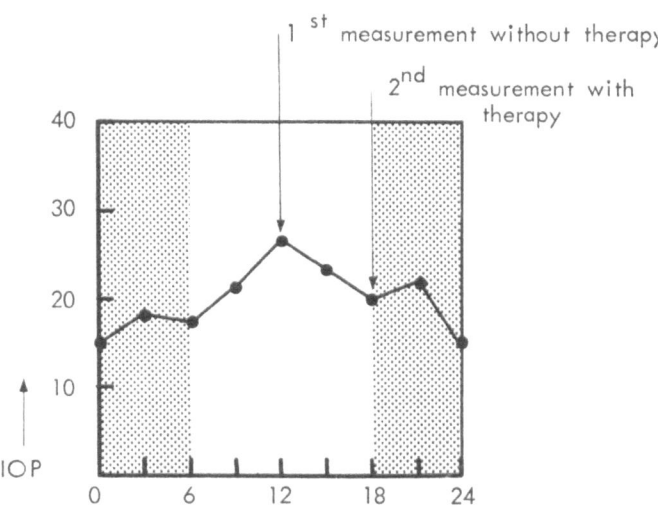

Fig. 4. Demonstration of a pseudo-effect of therapy in a patient that has his highest IOP without therapy at 12 o'clock. There is a fall of the IOP of approximately 5 mm. in the afternoon in the untreated patient. If the first measurement without therapy on day I has been made at 12 o'clock and the 2nd measurement with therapy on day II at 6 o'clock, a wrong impression of effectiveness of therapy is given.

119

only takes his eyedrops before he goes to the doctor and normally takes them at irregular intervals. In general it is better to discuss with the patient the time of the day in which he shall take his eye-drops than to prescribe eye-drops four times a day and leave it to the patient when he takes his drops). In both cases we can change our therapy in such a way that a 24 hour control of IOP can be expected. If there is progression of the visual field at constant low IOP levels other factors must be involved. In these unfortunate case it is often very difficult to stop the progression.

If the progression of the visual field took place at intermediate levels of IOP the same questions can be asked as for the low levels. If there are no peaks of the IOP at night and the patient takes his medication regularly we have to reduce the IOP further. Then we start the same order of events as after the original therapeutic test series.

Is it really necessary to evaluate our therapeutic regimes in such an elaborate way? The answer of course is yes. Glaucoma is a slowly progressive disease that may ultimately end in blindness. If we want to prevent this deplorable ultimate stage of glaucoma and we want to start a regime of *years of medical therapy* that may greatly effect the patient's personal life, we have to be sure that our regime really does what it is supposed to do. Once we are through this first circumstantial stage of evaluation we can control the patient at longer intervals.

Level of IOP with therapy

In the case of a glaucoma suspect where there are no visual field defects and there are no other risk factors present, one is usually content if the IOP can be reduced to the low twenties. Of course this again is an arbitrary level. But we do not know what the critical IOP of this patient is and we do not want to bother him with too heavy therapeutic regimes, as long as he has no visual field defects.

In the case of the established glaucoma patient with visual field defects the requirements for reduction of IOP are much more stringent. In general one can say that the greater the damage of visual function, the lower the IOP has to be. The ideal situation would be if the IOP could be reduced to levels of the low teens. Ultimately the effectiveness of therapy can only be based on comparative visual field examination. An IOP range around 20 mm in established glaucoma is no reason for satisfaction. Only if the visual field remains unchanged with this IOP range the therapy is sufficient.

Choice of the drug

In the preceeding papers all the drugs that are presently available for the treatment of glaucoma have been discussed. In the vast majority of cases the first drug to be used is pilocarpine or a similar miotic.If these miotic agents do not have a satisfactory effect or have undesirable side-effects one could also use epinephrine as the first and only medication. Epinephrine may also be useful in patients who have a cataract in order to avoid miosis. As a routine we use pilocarpine in different concentrations, aceclidine and sometimes carbachol. Epinephrine is used frequently. If necessary and possible we try to combine epinephrine with guanethidine. We have seen impressive reductions of IOP with a combination of a miotic, epinephrine and guanethidine. Even diamox can be added to this regime.

We do use diamox for long-term treatment of certain patients. In some instances eserine and mintacol may be useful. In aphakics phospholine iodide can be used.

The more therapeutic agents we use however, the smaller the chance that the patient will be able to take his medicins on the long run.

The system of prescribing pilocarpine once a day in case of dubiously raised IOP must be discouraged because it is too little therapy for a glaucoma patient and too much therapy for a healthy eye.

Unsatisfactory reduction of IOP

In some cases the prescribed medicin does not work. It is known that miotics can give *in 5%* of the cases a paradox rise of IOP. This can happen in simple glaucoma with a narrow angle, in cases with a increased size of the ageing lens, in the case of plateau iris, and in haemorrhagic glaucoma. Also after lens-extraction such paradox rises of IOP have been described. In cases of narrow angle glaucoma an angle closure can be precipitated by the use of miotics and not so infrequently.

It is known that medical therapy does not usually work in buphthalmus, in aniridia, in dysgenesis mesodermalis, in essential atrophy of the iris and in haemorrhagic glaucoma.

Antiglaucomatous drugs may loose their effect after a certain period of treatment. Therefore if the IOP rises under therapy it is important to stop the drug to see whether it still has the desired effect on IOP. Often the IOP shows again a good reaction to the drug after a period of withdrawal. If during the treatment with a certain agent the IOP slowly rises this can be due to the adaption to the drug, but it can also be due to progression of the disease. True progression, that is a rise of the baseline IOP, can be recognized by comparing the present IOP without therapy with the first measurements of IOP without therapy.

DRUG WARNINGS (APPENDIX)

Numerous drugs commonly used systemicaly in general medicin carry a warning against their use in patients with glaucoma. Most of these medications are para—sympatholytic agents or other agents that might produce pupillary dilatation. Unless they are used in near toxic doses there is little evidence that these drugs will adversely effect IOP in patients on therapy for primary open angle glaucoma. Such drugs can be potentially dangerous in the patient with an anatomically narrow angle and may precipitate an attack of angle closure glaucoma. Patients with known angle closure glaucoma should have had bilateral iridectomies that would prevent angle closure from mydriasis. Since open angle glaucoma is not adversely affected and angle closure glaucoma after iridectomy is not affected the only patient in potential danger is one who has undiagnosed angle closure glaucoma. When questioned before administration of a drug he of course would not know that he has glaucoma. For the most part therefore drug warnings concerning glaucoma are of little value except for medical legal protection of the manifacturer (Havener, 1974).

REFERENCES AND RECOMMENDED LITERATURE

Bigger, J.F. Comparison of the patient compliance is treated vs. untreated ocular hypertension. *Trans. Amer. Acad. Ophthal. 81,277*, (1976).

Drance, S.M. Medical management of early chronic open angle glaucoma. Symposium on glaucoma; Trans. New. Orleans. Acad. Ophthal; Mosby, St. Louis, 1975.

Drance, S.M. The significance of the diurnal tension variations in normal and glaucomatous eyes. *Arch. Ophthal. 64, 494*, (1960).

Goldmann, H. An analysis of some concepts concerning chronic simple glaucoma. *Amer. J. Ophthal. 80, 409*, 1975.

Greve, E.L. Single and multiple stimulus static perimetry in glaucoma; the two phases of visual field examination. *Docum. Ophthal. 36, 1-355*, (1973).

Greve, E.L. & Verduin, W. Detection of early glaucomatous damage. Proc. of the 2nd Int. Visual Field Symposium 1976. Junk B.V., the Hague. To be published 1977.

Greve, E.L. 'Perimetry' in 'Glaucoma: Pathogenesis, Diagnosis, Therapy'. Heilmann, K, Richardson, K., editors. Thieme, Stuttgart. To be published 1977.

Hager, H. Die Behandlung des Glaukoms mit Miotica. Bucherei des Augenartzes Heft 29, 1958.

Havener, W.M. Ocular pharmacology. Mosby, St. Louis, 1974.

Phelps, C.D. & Phelps, G.K. Measurement of Intra-ocular Pressure: study of its reproducibility. *Graefes Arch. Ophthal. 198, 39*, 1976.

Schaffer, R.N. 'Gonioscopy'. Symposium on glaucoma. Trans. New. Orleans. Acad. Opthal; Mosby, St.Louis, 1975.

Wilenski, J.T. & Podos, S.M. Prognostic parameters in primary open angle glaucoma. Symposium on glaucoma. Trans. New. Orleans. Acad. Ophthal; Mosby, St.Louis, 1975.

Author's address:
Eye Clinic of the University of Amsterdam
Wilhelmina Gasthuis
Eerste Helmerstraat 104
Amsterdam
The Netherlands

MEDICAL VERSUS SURGICAL THERAPY IN GLAUCOMA PATIENTS

R. SMITH

(London)

I should like first to make a few remarks about the medical treatments in current use in the Glaucoma Clinic at Moorfields, City Road, and then to describe to you an attempt to gain a little more knowledge of raised intra-ocular pressure on the visual fields.

I have little new to say on the subject of medical therapy. We tend to use Pilocarpine as our main stand-by, normally in 2%, 4% or sometimes 6% concentration. The commonest frequency of administration is three times daily, but many patients are on it more frequently.

In the last few weeks we have obtained a supply of Ocuserts delivering 40 micrograms of Pilocarpine. These can be left in the conjunctival sac for one week and are claimed to reduce the side effects which come from variations in myopia and pupillary size.

First impressions are that the device is well tolerated, but it is too early for us to say whether the advantages are big enough to justify the probable high price.

When patients are not adequately controlled on Pilocarpine, the tendency is to try other drugs before resorting to surgery. We use Neutral Adrenaline 1% twice daily, and in some cases this is preceded by a drop of Guanethidine 5%, ten minutes before. In a proportion of cases, quite spectacular results are achieved (Romano, 1974). Eserine is used in a few cases: some patients seem to be able to tolerate it as long term therapy, contrary to expectations. Tosmilen is used in a few cases as is prostigmine and occasionally pholine iodide. Long-term diamox in doses of 125 mg. twice daily or more is well tolerated by relatively few patients, the majority finding the side effects troublesome. We do not find daranide any better than diamox and it is rarely used in our clinic.Both are absolutely contra-indicated if renal pain is encountered or if one eye has a satisfactory surgical draining-bleb — I regard this as very important.

I find the results of medical treatment to be variable and erratic and suspect that this may be due to great variations in absorption of the various drugs from time to time, together with inexplicable changes in IOP in spite of treatment. I feel that one of our great defects in glaucoma management is the lack of some device by which IOP could be continuously monitored and even better, recorded. However many times we take the IOP — either in so-called attempts at phasing or on numerous clinic visits at varying times of the day, nevertheless these readings are but a minute sample of what is happening day by day over months and years. Even if we took the IOP a hundred times in a year we would only be monitoring this variable factor for an infinitesimal part of the time, and from what I have to say later you will see that this is indeed a very serious defect in our assessment of the situation.

I should now like to turn to my second subject, a study of the relationship between raised IOP and visual field loss.

It would be very valuable to be able to predict, in a given case, what was the probability of further substantial progression of visual field loss. At present we have little information on this. We are not able to say that an average IOP of say 21 mm. Hg. is safe, whereas 24 mm Hg. is not, since we all know of cases which by no means follow such a rigid rule. Several authors, for example, Armaly (1964) Drance (1962) and Goldmann (1972) have attempted to devise tests of susceptibility based on artificial elevation of IOP and its observed effect on field, but these have so far not reached a sufficiently refined stage to be reliable. It is not even easy to prove that IOP per se does cause field loss although it seems obvious that it must do so.

With these problems in mind I now turn to my long-term follow-up of cases of glaucoma simplex at Moorfields, which has now been running for almost twelve years.

I won't bore you with anything but the barest details of the study which has been published elsewhere, Smith (1972), but just remind you that I have been studying a group of approximately fifty patients with glaucoma simplex at three monthly intervals of whom half were randomised for a surgical operation (Scheie) at the outset, the other half acting as controls and remaining on medical treatment.

All sorts of problems arose however, — the timing of surgery was not uniform — for various reasons it was delayed and in some patients for up to a year. An increasing proportion of the so-called medical group eventually had operations, on unavoidable clinical grounds so that this single group split into two groups each subject to selection — the non-operated being ipso-facto those who had done best and who hence presumably would have had a better prognosis anyway.

Thus crude comparison of the two groups for the whole of their follow-up periods is now by no means a comparison between a surgically treated as

TABLE 1.

Pressures: Medical — Unoperated vs. Surgical — Operated

Years:		1	2	3	4	5	6	7	8	9	10	
Medical												
Mean I.O.P.	26:	24	23	22	24	22	26	23	26	24	22	Mean Medical
N	26:	22	20	15	11	11	6	6	4	3	2	23.6
Surgical												
Mean I.O.P.	25:	14	14	15	16	16	15	17	17	18	16	Mean Surgical
N	25:	21	24	23	21	20	16	13	8	5	2	15.8
Differences												
Medical —												Mean
Surgical:		10	9	7	8	6	11	6	9	6	6	differences
												7.8
												P < .001

124

opposed to a medically treated group. It is on the other hand a comparison between two initially randomised (and comparable) groups, one of which had an arbitrary decision for early surgery and the other which had what one might call a conventional routine — that is to say surgery delayed as long as possible. Thus the eventual distinction between the two groups is much less sharp than one had hoped for in the first place.

However, I have all the facts — three monthly pressures, acuities and visual field scores (on a percentage basis) for all the patients, and it is possible therefore to try and find correlations of one sort or another which might be meaningful.

RESULTS

If we try and see what has been happening to these cases it might be helpful to look at the IOP first. Table 1 shows the IOP in all surgical cases which had an operation versus all medical which had not.

It can be seen at once that there is a clear advantage for surgery in terms of IOP; the mean IOP difference being 7.8 mm. Hg. with a high significance level.

What we now have to find out is whether we can demonstrate that this 'pressure advantage' does any good to our patients. If we study only the cases referred to in the IOP study — that is the randomised surgical cases who had actually ondergone surgery and the randomised medical cases who had not undergone surgery, our analysis is to a certain extent biased by selection. The 'medical' group although initially containing all the randomised medical cases was gradually reduced in numbers by the removal of unfavourable cases which were forced to have surgery because they were not doing well. For example at year four there were 21 'surgicals' but the 'medicals' had been reduced to eleven. The tendency would be for the medical group gradually to alter its nature as time went on; the proportion of favourable to unfavourable cases within the group rising as the unfavourable cases were removed due to their being operated upon. By year 4, for example, 10 'medical' cases had been removed and of the remaining 11 only 3 later needed surgery — 8 did not. Thus by this time the 'medical' group was heavily weighted with favourable cases. The effect of this would presumably be to mask possible beneficial effects of surgery in the 'surgical' as opposed to the 'medical' group.

If we now study the fate of the visual fields in these patients it is apparent that this is exactly what does happen since the actual pooled field scores show only a slight advantage to the surgical group throughout the ten year period, in spite of the built-in statistical disadvantage of the surgical group (Fig. 1).

The mean advantage in visual field score of the surgical group over the medical over the whole ten year period is only 5.2 however, and by the student T test thus is not a significant difference. But we have to bear in mind that the two groups are no longer fully comparable (Table 2).

There is one rather important and disturbing corollary to these figures. If in fact the 'surgical' group did as well as or little better than the unoperated 'medicals' this means that approximately half of those patients (the equi-

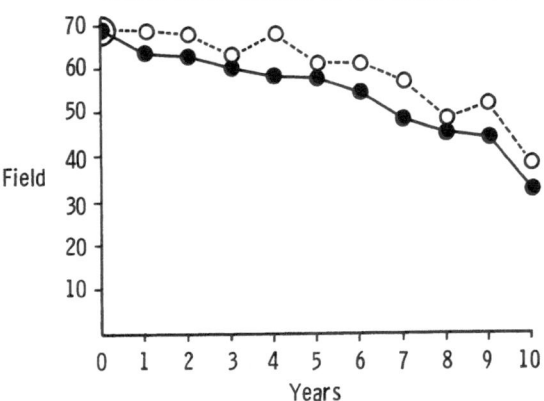

Differences between Pooled Field Scores

Surgical (Operated) and Medical (Unoperated)

Fig. 1.

TABLE 2.

Pooled Visual Field Scores,

Medical (Unoperated) vs. Surgical (Operated)

Years·		1	2	3	4	5	6	7	8	9	10	
Medical												
Mean Field	69:	64	64	61	58	58	56	49	46	46	34	Mean 53.6
N	27:	24	19	13	11	11	7	6	4	3	2	
Surgical												
Mean Field	66:	69	68	63	69	61	61	56	49	53	39	Mean 58.8
N	26:	21	23	24	22	20	18	14	10	6	2	
Differences												
Medical −												Mean
Surgical:		5	4	2	11	3	5	7	3	7	5	differences 5.2
												$P < 0.3$ i.e. N/S

valent ones to the favourable 'medicals') need never have been operated upon. The trouble is that at present we are unable to identify which cases had the 'unnecessary' operations.

It would probably be best at this point to confine our attention for a moment to the 'medical' cases during their pre-operative period — this group is a representative sample of glaucoma simplex under pure medical therapy and contains patients showing varying rates of field deterioration. Can we correlate this field deterioration with IOP?

First therefore let us look at the correlation between IOP and field score in these cases. The method of studying this has been to determine the regression of field score against time in each of such cases and to compare these regression with the IOP. Table 3 shows all these regressions together with the mean IOP over the follow-up period of each case (taking only cases with a follow-up of five years or more).

It can be seen that there is poor correlation between the behaviour of the fields and the mean IOP over this period. r = .4419; p < .2 (not significant).

To sum up the position so far; we have shown that surgery undoubtedly

TABLE 3.   Medical: mean IOP's

IOP	Field
28.39	− 5.88
27.34	− 4.13
23.26	− 4.17
24.82	− 1.10
22.09	− 2.48
24.38	− 1.14
21.5	− 3.18
19.56	− 5.15
19.42	− 1.93
19.78	+ 0.41
MX = 23.54	MY = 2.875
r = −.4419	p < .2 (N/S)

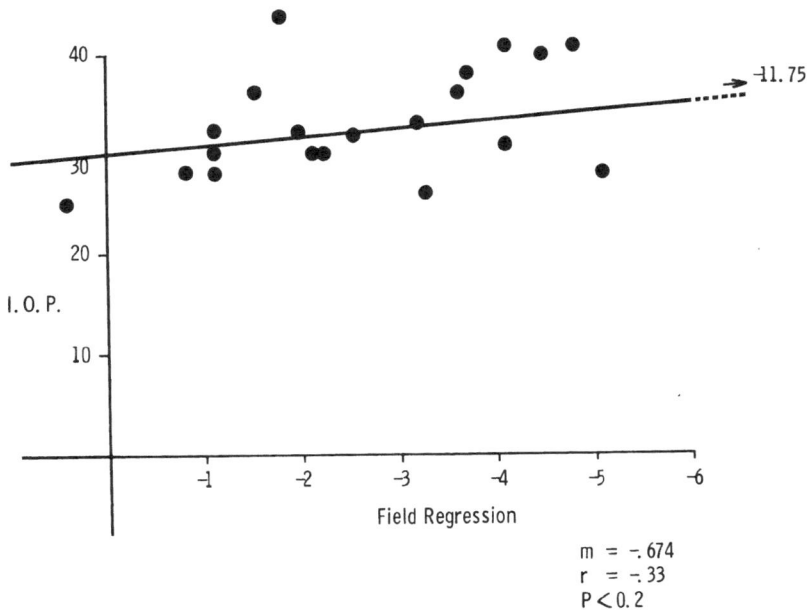

MEDICAL CASES

I.O.P.

Field Regression

m = −.674
r = −.33
P < 0.2

Fig. 2.

lowers IOP better than medical therapy. We have shown that there is a possible slight advantage in terms of rate of field loss in operated as compared to unoperated cases, but we have not been able to prove, in unoperated medical cases that field progression is related to raised IOP.

A further attempt to extract from our figures some correlation of field change with IOP now seems imperative. Accordingly the next thing we shall look at is the behaviour of all the 'medical' cases. If we again tabulate them as in Table 3 we find there is again poor correlation between field deterioration and the average IOP of each case over the period. But we can do something a little different. We can assume that below some critical IOP (which we cannot identify) no harm is done to the field. Harm can only come above this IOP. So if we now plot the field regressions against the highest single IOP recorded during the period for each case we may find some correlation. The plot is shown in Fig. 2 and shows a correlation of $-.33$ with a trend of $-.674$ per mm. Hg. But again it is not statistically significant.

This is disappointing but if we pause for a moment we can think of an explanation. The group contains a large proportion (about half) of patients who had had an operation at some time during their career. Hence the highest IOP in those people usually occurred pre-operatively and several years of low IOP would follow – so that the single high IOP would not be expected to be in character for that patient for much of the period of study.

As a final attempt to relate field deterioration to IOP let us turn to the 'surgical' group. Again we have calculated all the regressions of field score on time for these patients. The regressions we have taken here are those field scores occurring after the surgery. We have calculated these regressions against the mean IOP of the surgical cases post-operatively and we find that field score correlates with pressure to the extent of $-.526$, again not a very strong correlation but nevertheless significant $p < .01$.

But now comes the really exciting part – if we ignore the pre-operative IOP and the first post-operative IOP (in the first three months), and pick out the highest IOP in each case recorded subsequently we can tabulate them as per Table 4, and Fig. 3.

We see now that the field deterioration correlates better with IOP and that the rate of field loss escalates by -1.2 per annum per mm. Hg. increment of IOP. The result seems to support the view that IOP as such is damaging to visual fields – a concept which everyone was aware of already but about which definite evidence has hitherto been lacking.

My reading of the picture is as follows – in any given case the mean IOP is of little importance since it may be weighted with numerous normal readings and these normal readings indicate periods during which no damage occurs. What matters to the patient is the amount of pressure-time he has above damage level, the high intra-ocular-pressure dose in fact. If you look at it like the damaging effects of a cumulative drug, his periods of normal IOP do him little or no positive good – his periods of high IOP do him irreversible harm.

If we could now begin to assess the sort of high pressures – time dose which is going to do significant damage, we might be in a better position to form judgments as to the fate of the patient.

Although taking only one IOP reading as characteristic of each individual seems to be making rather a sweeping assumption about what happens during all the rest of the time, nevertheless, I think it is justified. It shows that the eye in question has the capability of producing very high IOP and as such it stigmatises that eye as being dangerous. Another individual might

TABLE 4.   Surgical post-OP

IOP	Field
19	− 2.52
22	− 9.3
22	− 1.87
21	0.5
24	− 1.7
25	− 2.1
22	− 5.1
24	− 5.7
28	− 0.547
18	.714
31	− 8.59
22	− 0.857
19	− 0.428
21	− 2.285
18	2.075
10	1.742
20	1.657
27	− 2.68
22	− 3.542
32	− 6.00
MY = 22.35	MX = 2.07
r = −.526	p < .01

SURGICAL CASES: POSTOPERATIVE PERIOD

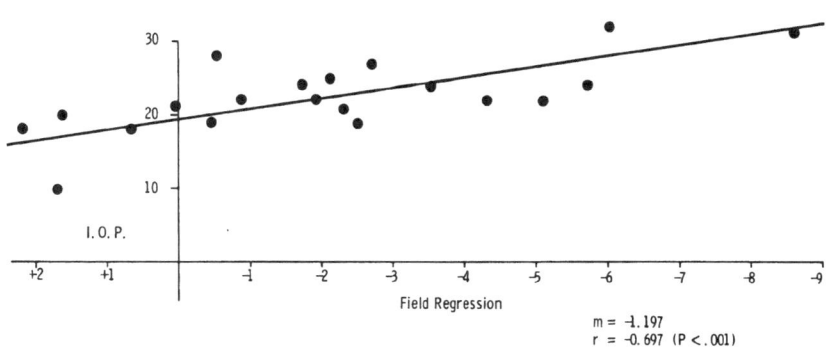

m = −1.197
r = −0.697 (P < .001)

Fig. 3.

even show a higher than average IOP but not such high peaks. Thus his total dose of high IOP time is likely to be less.

In summary therefore I have attempted to show that our continuing assessment of medical control based on sample IOP readings tends to be very ineffective in the absence of any method of continuous recording of pressure. Nevertheless I have been able to show that raised IOP does indeed correlate with increasing field loss so that our efforts to keep IOP pressure down to a minimum are eminently justified.

REFERENCES

Armaly, M. Topical Dexamethasone application. *Arch. Ophthal.* 71, *636* (1964).
Drance, S. Studies in the susceptibility of the eye to raised intra-ocular pressure. *Trans. Ophthal. Soc. U.K.*, 82, *73* (1962).
Goldmann, H. Open Angle Glaucoma (Symposium) *Brit. J. Ophthal.* 56, *242* (1972).
Romano, J. In Discussion. *Trans. Ophthal. Soc. U.K.* 94, *576* (1974).
Smith, R.J.H. Medical versus Surgical Therapy in Glaucoma Simplex. *Brit. J. Ophthal.* 56, *277* (1972).

Author's address:
2 Harley Street
London WIN IAA
England

DISCUSSION

Chairman: E.L. Greve

Greve:

Ladies and gentlemen, we now proceed to answering some questions that have been asked by the audience. I shall start immediately with a question to one of the Paterson's and the question is: Is there any risk of cataract after the treatment with guanethidine and let us extend the question, any risk of cataract after a treatment with any of the adrenergic drugs?

Mrs. Paterson:

I think the answer to that is 'No'. We have not found any evidence of cataract in any of our patients on this drug.

Greve:

Then a question has been asked whether it is advisable to use a combination of pilocarpine and eserine and I think that it has been answered already in one of our speeches. The answer was that it does not make much sense to use this combination.

Now an important question: What are the possibilities for regulation of the IOP at night; the common therapy of four times pilocarpine a day probably does not cut off the peak-pressures and as we have just heard from Redmond Smith the peak-pressures may very well be those pressures that cause deterioration of the field, Klaus could you comment on that?

Heilmann:

Redmond Smith's paper was very interesting for me. If his interpretation of the role of peak-pressures for the progression of visual field defects in glaucoma is correct, the consequence has to be a constant diurnal pressure level. In the conservative treatment constancy in IOP only can be achieved by constant intraocular tissue levels of a pressure reducing substance. This only can be by constant achieved by a Therapeutic System with a zero-order drug release kinetic, e.g. Ocusert-Pilocarpine with a functional life time of one week.

Greve:

Drance has shown that 8% pilocarpine has an effect of 8 hours on IOP and that it could be used for controlling the night IOP peaks.

Then another question that came up is this: Are there at present drugs that have a good pressure-lowering effect, but intolerable side-effects, that could be used effectively in a lower concentration, e.g. in systems for sustained release. Could I ask that question to one of the Paterson's. Probably some of the adrenergic drugs might be used in membrane.

Mr. Paterson

I think that iso-prenaline might be a possibility here, because when you give it in a large concentration it gets absorbed systemically. If you could administer it in smaller amounts continuously, you might well get good control. Drance did try to reduce his concentration of iso-prenaline but of course the moment he lost his tachycardia he also lost his effect on IOP, but the Ocusert might be an answer to this.

Greve:

I think Gillian Paterson also suggested using Ocusert for the reduction of the concentration of adrenaline?

Mrs. Paterson:

No, guanethidine.

Greve:

Then a question about the additive effects of adrenergic drugs. We have now heard about additive affects of adrenaline and guanethidine. Could any of the other drugs effectively be used in combination, e.g. bèta-blockers.

Mr. Paterson:

Well, certainly, I know that Drance did try iso-prenaline applied locally with propanolol applied systemically. The idea there was that you would block the effects of tachycardia, but not effect the actions of iso-prenaline on the eye. So far as I know, no-one has tried the combination of adrenaline and bèta-blockers locally. We shall certainly have to wait to see what happens then.

Mrs. Paterson:

I have a few patients who have been very difficult to control and I have added Propanolol systemically to their regime which had included adrenaline and succeeded in dropping the IOP by another 4-5 mm. Less than half a dozen patients, but that does seem to be an effect on the top of the effect produced by adrenaline.

Greve:

Rob, do you have any experiences.

Brenkman:

I can agree with you. We had in our investigation into the effect of Practolol eye-drops, also patients who were not very well regulated on a combination of pilocarpine and adrenaline-like drugs and the addition of Practolol eye-drops showed in many patients a good effect. Not as strong as in the, let us say, fresh glaucoma-patients, but we found an effect.

Greve:

Then there is a question about the use of Catapresan or Clonidine. Klaus Heilmann has an experience with this drug and carried out investigations on this subject. Could you comment on that Klaus.

Heilmann:

Clonidine is a very interesting pharmacological substance and a problematic drug as well. Clonidine lowers elevated and normal intraocular pressure, the reduction can occur after local or systemic application. Local application of the substance produces dose dependent systemic side-effects: dryness of the mouth, sedation, bradycardia and a fall in blood pressure. This latter effect may be hazardous. In animals it was shown that the substance neither improves outflow facility nor inhibits aqueous formation but shows marked intraocular vasoconstriction (Bill & Heilmann 1975). A fall in blood pressure and vasoconstriction in the arterioles supplying the optic nerve head may reduce blood flow even if IOP is reduced. This is the problem and the danger.

If we talk about Clonidine we also should talk about epinephrine. We have heard something today about epinephrine bur a very important aspect is usually missing in the discussion of its side effects. The fact that adrenergic substances are extremely vasoactive is not sufficiently taken into account. After an intracutanous injection of a few microgrammes of epinephrine very strong vasoconstriction results in the region of the injection, kidney filtration is reduced under epinephrine treatment, higher doses reduce the filtration rate by the contraction of the vas afferens. The kidney is a vital organ, protected to a great extent by regulatory mechanisms; up till now the existence of similar protecting mechanisms for the optic nerve have not been found. If elevated IOP causes damage to the optic nerve head by limiting its blood supply, then every reduction of IOP will improve the circulatory situation. This presupposes, however, that the pressure-reducing agent does not simultaneously act on the circulation. And here I think is the real problem for epinephrine: its vascular effects in the eye and possible further effects on the blood supply to the optic nerve are to a great extent unknown. In the patient's interest epinephrine and its derivatives should not be used uncritically for the treatment of glaucoma.

Greve:

I think we have heard from Gillian Paterson that epinephrine can be used in lower concentrations than we usually do. In this 5-year follow-up study of guanethidine and adrenaline did you find any development of defects or deterioration of defects?

Mrs. Paterson:

No, the 5-year numbers were small, 10-15 and they have been controlled in every sense of the word.

Greve:

Then a question about the use of Thymoxamine. Gillian, can you say something about that?

Mrs. Paterson:

This drug has been used by some workers. I know for certain that Etienne in Lyon has used it in the treatment of narrow-angle and closed-angle glaucoma and its use lies in the fact that it is quite a powerful miotic agent. It is an adrenergic alpha-blocking agent and it acts by blocking the sympathetically inervated dilator of the pupil. It leaves the sphincter unopposed and the miosis with a 0.1% solution is intense. It comes on within half an hour and lasts up to 2-3 hours if the strength is increased up to 1% a miosis lasting up to 48 hours can be produced. 1% Thymoxamine is not very comfortable; it is a painful drop to instill, but it is being used by some workers for the treatment of the acute attack of angle-closure glaucoma.

Greve:

There is a question here and maybe Leo Dake can answer that; it is about the risk of cataract and iriscysts in long treatment of strabismic children with phospholine iodide.

Dake:

Iris-cysts in children have been described after the use of irreversible cholinesterase inhibitors. To my knowledge there is one publication about 10 years ago about a reversible cataract in a child treated with phospholine iodide for strabismus. As a last comment: I should not like to have my children treated with phospholine iodide for strabismus.

Greve:

From the talk of Redmond Smith I got the impression that patients are, as far as their pressures are concerned, better of with surgical treatment than with medical treatment. Who wants to comment the following question:

Does medical therapy prevent deterioration of glaucoma and if not, is this because it is not taken adequately, because of the mechanism of action, because it does not reduce the IOP adequately, because of high pressures at night, or any other reason? Peter Graham, could you comment on that.

Graham:

Well, I think in many cases medical therapy fails therepautically and not pharmacologically because, as has been repeated many times to-day, it is one thing to prescribe a treatment for a patient and it is another thing to have him follow the prescribed treatment-regime. Some of the failures of medical therapy are due not to the pharmacological inactivity of the drugs that we prescribe, but to the fact that the patient is not using them. But having said that I think there is little doubt that in many patients medical therapy does fail and that one can get a greater reduction of IOP with probably less lability of IOP at times when we may not detect them, by surgical treatment. This comes back to what Redmond Smith was just saying. Maybe surgical treatment is less liable to peaks of IOP and even at the same mean IOP is therefore a more reliable means of control.

Greve:

Redmond, any further comments on this matter.

Smith:

Well, only just to reinforce what Klaus Heilmann said and that is that it seems to me that if in fact inconstancy of pressure peaks are what we should really be worrying about rather than main pressure (and especially this applies to pressure at night or very early in the morning before the patient has taken the drops) that the Ocusert might be much better than the conventional course of drops-therapy, if it could produce a more even level-pressure, even if it was 22 or 23 with guaranteed no peaks.

Heilmann:

We have a long follow-up study of patients treated with Ocusert-Pilocarpine. We perform once a month an IOP day-curve and see that the IOP are regulated. The IOP variations between morning and afternoon are about 2-3mm Hg. This variation is in the range of physiological diurnal variation of IOP.

Brenkman:

Perhaps I can comment on the subject of the peaks. We have used the water-drinking provocation test to get information about possible peak-IOP. We have performed the test before and after the administration of a bèta-blocking drug (10% practolol eye drops) in a patient with a serious juvenile glaucoma. We noticed a great difference in the effect of the water-drinking test on the IOP with and without therapy. The peak-IOP was much higher without therapy, so in this case we know that the patient was safe with respect to his peak-IOP, using these eye drops.

Greve:

I wish to thank all the participants in the discussion. We have now reached the end of this symposium. I can assure you that we had many more subjects, many more questions, but I think we have taken too much of your patience, patience not of your patients, and we would like to leave it at that. As one conclusion I should like to say that I think that in the field of medical therapy in glaucoma there are some highly interesting developments and that on the one hand we have the controlled delivery systems, which are very promising indeed, and that on the other hand there are the adrenergic drugs that are in stage of great development at the moment.

We would like to thank you all very much for your presence and hope that you enjoyed the day.

SUMMARY

E.L. GREVE & C.L. DAKE

(Amsterdam)

On the cholinergic side of medical therapy in glaucoma, pilocarpine, aceclidine and carbachol are the well-known and widely used drugs. New developments are not in the drugs but in the controlled delivery by means of membrane systems as, for instance, pilocarpine-Ocusert. Such systems for continuous zero-order release of drugs can be used for any eye-drops. Their main advantages are: avoidance of the overdose-underdose regime; lower quantities of drug possible; better control of night IOP; avoidance of the psychological effects of a QID eyedrop regime.

The adrenergic therapeutic field has widened considerably. The combination of epinephrine and guanethidine is usefull and potent. Some of the β-blocking drugs may well be a valuable aid to non-miotic therapy. More developments are expected in this area.

As far as the clinical management of the glaucoma is concerned the following statements can be given:

— the patient is not afraid of a raised IOP but of loss of visual function.

— exact relation between IOP and visual function i.e. the critical IOP is unknown in a glaucoma suspect.

— the beginning of therapy in a glaucoma *suspect* depends on an evaluation of the base-line IOP, risk factors and possible side-effects of therapy.

— an arbitrary level of 25 mm to 30 mm is usually accepted as the level above which therapy has to be initiated in a glaucoma suspect.

— in an *established* glaucoma patient there is no doubt that therapy has to be started; the aim is to reach IOP levels around 15 mm or even lower.

— the evaluation of therapeutic effects is of primary importance and can best be done by means of diurnal curves and left-right comparison.

— the effect of therapy should be prevention of progression of field defects. Ultimately the follow-up visual field examinations give the answer whether a certain reduction of IOP is adequate or not.

— Redmond Smith concluded from his investigation that the peak IOP's are more damaging than the average IOP level.